Rehabilitation of Maxillofacial Defects with Prosthesis - An Outline

Pankaj Kharade

Rehabilitation of Maxillofacial Defects with Prosthesis- An Outline

LAP LAMBERT Academic Publishing

Imprint

Any brand names and product names mentioned in this book are subject to trademark, brand or patent protection and are trademarks or registered trademarks of their respective holders. The use of brand names, product names, common names, trade names, product descriptions etc. even without a particular marking in this work is in no way to be construed to mean that such names may be regarded as unrestricted in respect of trademark and brand protection legislation and could thus be used by anyone.

Cover image: www.ingimage.com

Publisher:
LAP LAMBERT Academic Publishing
is a trademark of
International Book Market Service Ltd., member of OmniScriptum Publishing Group
17 Meldrum Street, Beau Bassin 71504, Mauritius
Printed at: see last page
ISBN: 978-3-659-76086-0

Copyright © Pankaj Kharade
Copyright © 2015 International Book Market Service Ltd., member of OmniScriptum Publishing Group

Rehabilitation of Maxillofacial Defects with Prosthesis- A Concise summation

Author
Dr Pankaj Kharade

M.D.S., F.D.P.S.

Assistant Professor

Department of Prosthodontics

Dr Z A Dental College

Aligarh Muslim university

India.

INDEX

Introduction	2 – 3
Rehabilitation of Maxillary defect	4 –3 0
Rehabilitation of Mandibular defect	31 – 39
Rehabilitation of Tongue defect	40 – 43
Rehabilitation of Pharyngeal defect	44-52
Rehabilitation of Lip defect	53
Rehabilitation of Esophageal defect	54
Rehabilitation of Nasal defect	55
Rehabilitation of Orbital defect	56-65
Rehabilitation of Oculal defect	66-68
Rehabilitation of Auricular defect	69-73
Rehabilitation of Nasal defect	74
Rehabilitation of Nasal defect	75
Rehabilitation of Cranial defect	76
Discussion	77-78
Conclusion	79
References	80-90

Prosthetic Rehabilitation of Maxillofacial Defects – An Overview

Introduction-

The management of malignant tumors associated with the maxilla, tongue, floor of the mouth, mandible, and adjacent structures represents a difficult challenge for the oncosurgeon, radiation oncologist, and prosthodontist in accordance with both control of the primary disease and rehabilitation following surgical treatment. Disabilities resulting from such resections may include variety of situations such as impaired speech articulation, nasal regurgitation of fluids, difficulty in swallowing, problems with mastication, altered mandibular movements, compromised control of salivary secretions, and severe cosmetic disfigurement leading to altered psychological status as well as quality of life.

General guidelines for selecting treatment modality for oral cancer-

Stage I / II disease - Single modality (Surgery or Radiotherapy)

Stage III / IV disease - Combined modality

a. Surgery + Radiotherapy ± Chemotherapy
b. Chemotherapy + Radiotherapy

In case of surgical resection, most of the times it is not possible to reconstruct the post resection defect by surgical method. So prosthodontic rehabilitation of such patients is recommended to correct the structural, functional and esthetic disability. Patients who are undergoing radiation therapy are advised to undergo oral prophylaxis, extraction of grossly carious teeth, restoration of diseased teeth, replacement of missing teeth and topical fluoride application to prevent radiation induced caries. For patients undergoing chemotherapy same prophylactic dental treatment is indicated except topical fluoride application.

Rehabilitation of Maxillectomy patients-

Introduction-

Maxillary defects are the most frequent of all intraoral defects. The prosthesis used to close the maxillary defect is termed as obturator. Prosthetic rehabilitation with obturator or closure with microvascular free tissue flap are the treatment modalities following maxillectomy. Prosthetic rehabilitation bypasses many limitations of surgical treatment such as high treatment cost, surgical risk and its mental trauma. The obturator functions to keep the defect area clean, to reconstruct the palatal contour and/or soft palate, to improve speech or, to make speech possible. The most important objective of prosthodontic care emphasized by DeVan, is the preservation of remaining teeth and tissues. A comfortable cosmetically acceptable prosthesis that restores the impaired physiological objectives of speech, deglutition and mastication is a basic objective of prosthodontic care.

Obturators to correct acquired defects are basically of three types –

1. Immediate or surgical obturator
2. Interim obturator or Treatment or Transitional obturator
3. Definitive obturator

Immediate or Surgical obturator –

1. It supports the surgical packing in the resection cavity.
2. Restores continuity in the hard palate.

3. Restores the patients to take the oral nutrition.

   Dentulous /Edentulous surgical obturator should be secured by circumzygomatic wires, sutures or bone screws. Maxillary bones are used for wiring and sutures. Bone screws are placed through vomer. This obturator is inserted at the time of operation and removed after 5-10 days.

Interim obturator –

It restores deglutition and speech by restoring palatal contour by separating the nasal cavity from oral cavity. It remains for 2 to 12 weeks during the healing period.

Definitive Obturator-

It is fabricated and delivered after complete contracture leading to complete healing and remodelling of tissues. If teeth are preserved and properly distributed(close to or further away from the defect) retention and stability can be easily obtained by means of different parts of removable partial denture. The posterolateral region of the defect is used for proper sealing. So in presence of properly distributed teeth, obturator is not extended into defect area for retention and stability. In case of edentulous patients the obturator should be extended superior to the defect opening. Over extension into the defect along the nasal septum do not provide any stress bearing advantage as it is lined by pseudostratified columnar epithelium. Oral mucosa laterally and skin graft if found withstand more stresses from obturator and can be utilized. Superior extension of 8 to 10 mm into the defect area is adequate for stability and support. The cavity is convex from inferior to superior. At the height of convexity the cavity walls begin to turn towards the centre of the cavity. Superior aspect of the prosthesis should extend upto this point. Extension beyond this point would not provide any retention rather add to the weight of the prosthesis. Prosthesis may fall due to weight. Prosthesis should have some height for the passage of a liquid discharged between prosthesis and tissues to reach the oral cavity .The extended part should be hollow but closed to aid speech resonance, to lighten the weight of the prosthesis and to maintain facial aesthetics on the unsupported side of the obturator.

Definitive obturator with complete denture

Rehabilitation of completely edentulous maxillectomy defect is a very challenging procedure. Deficiency of retentive elements advocates for precise fabrication of maxillary complete denture with obturator. Hollowing of the bulb portion perk up the acceptance of the prosthesis due to lightened weight.

Initial step is to make primary impression in a most precise manner. Model is obtained from this impression and it is used for custom tray fabrication. With the help of custom tray the defect and its periphery are re-recorded and final impression is made in suitable impression material.

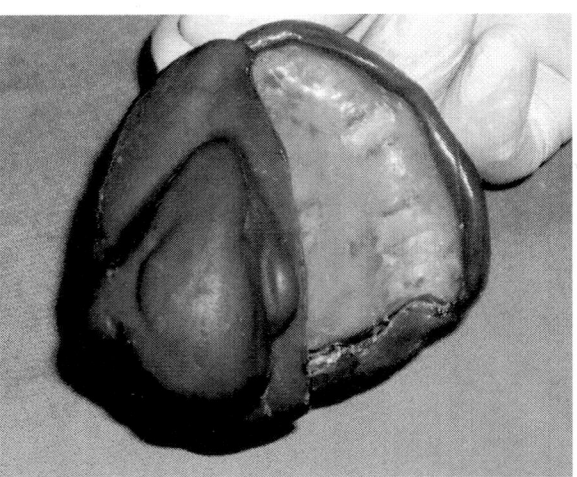

Fig- Impression of the intra oral defect

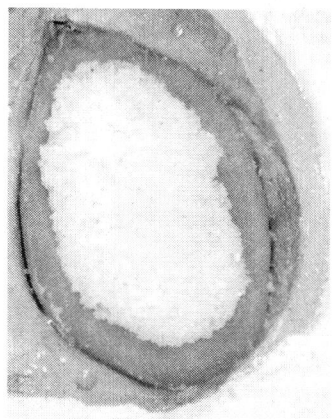

Fig- Defect portion filled with salt to make it hollow

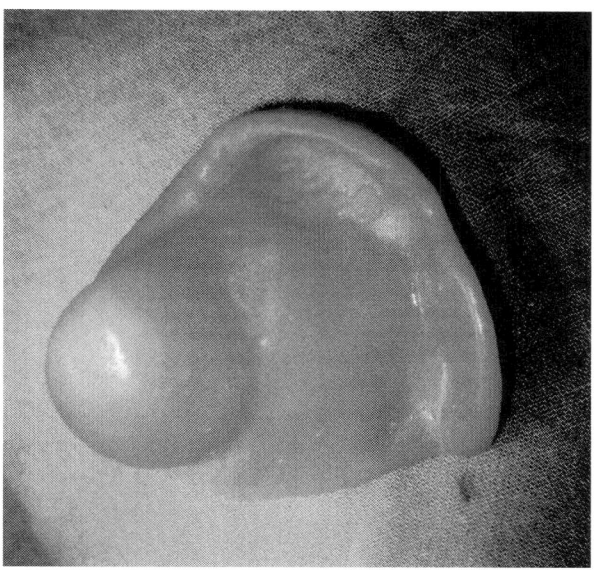

Fig- Final prosthesis with hollow bulb

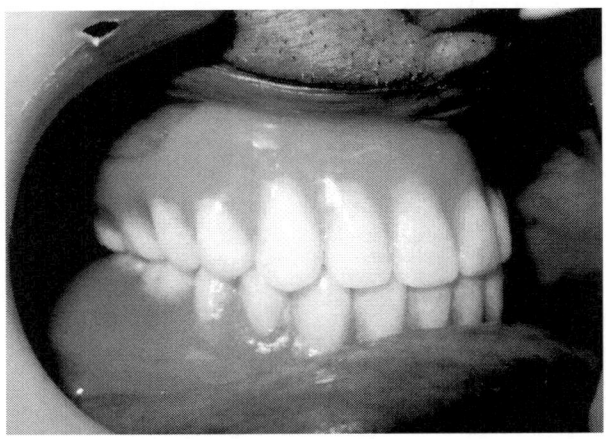

Fig- Final prosthesis in situ

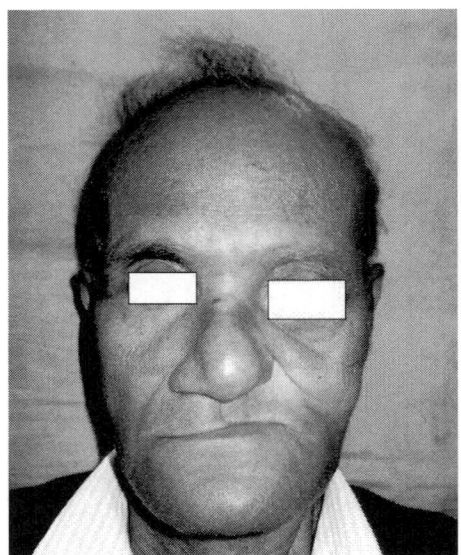

Fig- Before treatment

For larger defects hollowing techniques can be used to lighten the weight of the prosthesis. If salt is used to make the bulb hollow, it is later removed by making small hole and injecting water through it. After removal of salt the bulb portion is dried and sealed with autopolymerizing resin. The patient is instructed about use and maintenance of the prosthesis. Patient is advised for routine follow up and speech assessment session.

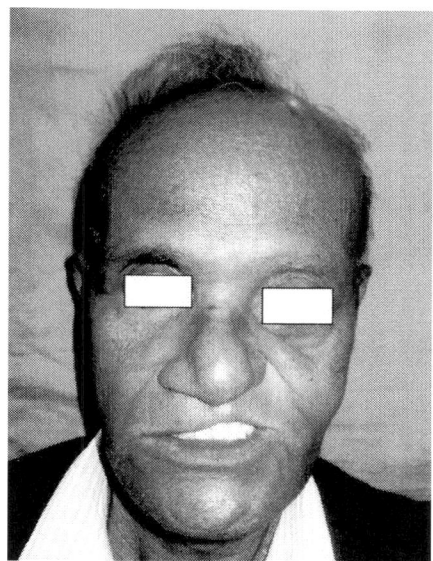

Fig- After treatment

Implant retained definitive obturator-

Implant retained definitive obturaor enhances the quality of life to a greater extent as implants provide additional retention. Additional retention is mostly needed in unusual cases such as large defects and totally edentulous maxilla. Eventhough implant retained prosthesis leads to excessive treatment cost, the treatment outcome is definitely satisfactory. Precise implant placement will minimize the difficulties encountered during the prosthesis fabrication.

After implant placement it is advisable to wait for 4-6 months depending on the quality of bone. In patients who have undergone radiotherapy placement of implants is usually delayed. All the clinical steps are carried out in same manner as for other definitive prosthesis. After fabrication of the final prosthesis, retentive components are fixed with the implants with its all components. Holes are prepared in the definitive prosthesis in accordance with location of the implants and retentive components which are supposed to be remain in the prosthesis are picked up with the help of autopolymerizing resin relining method. This method leads to precise placement of prosthesis on the implant attachments in the desired location and it minimizes unnecessary forces on the implants.

Masticatory performance and retention of the prosthesis is very much enhanced due to placement of implants. Such prostheses are very much useful from speech improvement point of view as well. Patient should be instructed for proper insertion and removal of the prosthesis so as to minimize maintenance problems with the implant attachments.

Difinitive prosthesis in maxilla grafted with free fibula flap

Maxillary defects created due to resection of the tumors in the maxilla are very difficult to restore. Apart from that these defects also lead to several problems like nasal regurgitation of food, speech articulation problem and difficulty in swallowing. If these defects are reconstructed and closure is achieved with the help of vascularised flaps such as free fibula graft, then all the above mentioned problems will get rectified. Reconstruction of maxilla with free fibula graft also provides option of rehabilitation with implant retained prosthesis as implant placement can be planned in the free fibula graft.

Fibula being a vascular bone very much favorable for osseointegration of implants. The composite fibular flap is nourished by the peroneal (fibular) vessels. The flap may be transferred with bone alone or with skin and muscle. The composite flap may include up to 25 cm of bone, more than 250 cm of lateral leg skin surface, a portion of the soleus muscle, and the entire flexor hallucis longus muscle if needed for complex defects. The bone's length and extensive periosteal blood supply allows the reconstruction of the resected mandible or maxilla. Multiple osteotomies may be performed to replicate the contour of the resected mandible without risk of devascularizing the bone segments. At least 6 cm of bone is left proximally and distally to maintain respective joint stability. The fibula's cortical nature and thickness make it an excellent recipient of osseointegrated implants, and the success rates appear to be quite good quality. Either leg may be utilized as a donor site, although the selection may be determined by the vascularity of the lower extremity, the side, location, and extent of the tumor resection, and the reconstructive surgeon's preference. When the ipsilateral neck is vessel depleted, the pedicle may be lengthened by using the distal bone and dissecting the periosteum.

Regular follow up is necessary for implant retained prosthesis in maxillary arch reconstructed with free fibula graft. Regular hygiene maintenance prevents flare ups of the soft tissues around the implants.

Definitive obturator prosthesis with Bar & Clip attachment

As surgery for such conditions is often radical, the prosthodontist is faced not only with the prosthodontic problems which are involved, but also the psychological problem of the patient's rehabilitation. In general, there is reduced capacity for residual teeth and tissue to provide optimal cross arch support, stability and retention. The design of the prosthesis must take into account the tooth-tissue support considerations and the impact of the altered environment on prosthesis support, stability and retention. Incorporation of Bar & Clip attachment in the definitive prosthesis helps to improve retention and stability of the prosthesis. Use of such attachments though leads to higher treatment cost, the treatment outcome is definitely enhanced and leads to improved quality of life.

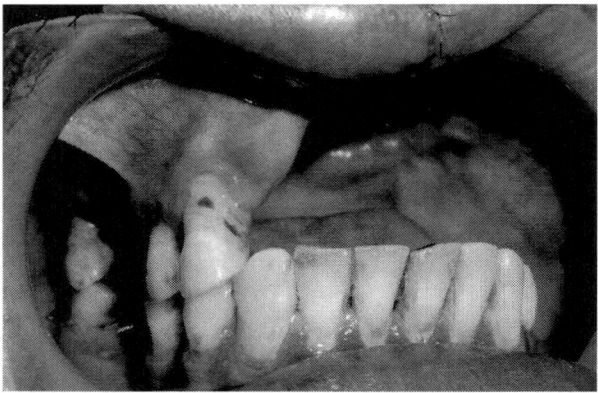

Fig- Maxillary defect with remaining teeth

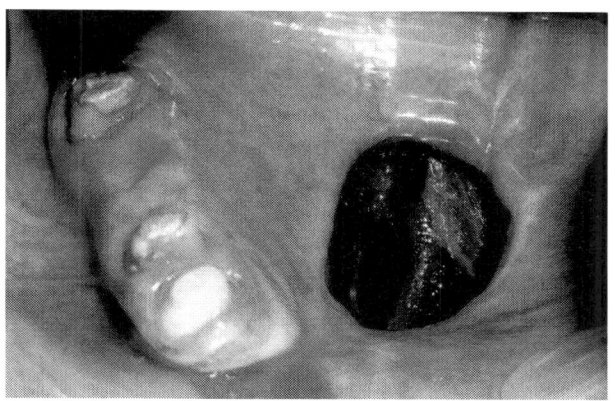

Fig- Crown preparation of remaining teeth done

Incorporation of bar is done by attaching the bar with the abutment copings during casting procedure. After crown preparation of the abutment teeth impressions are made and models are fabricated. The castable bar from the bar and clip attachment kit is attached with the wax pattern of the abutment copings. This entire unit is invested and casting procedure is carried out. After finishing and polishing this bar assembly is cemented in place and final impression of the maxillary defect along with the bar assembly is made. During packing and processing of the heat cure resin the defect portion is made hollow with the help of salt hollowing technique. The metal casings from the clip attachments are kept on the model replicating the bar portion. Later packing of heat cure resin and processing

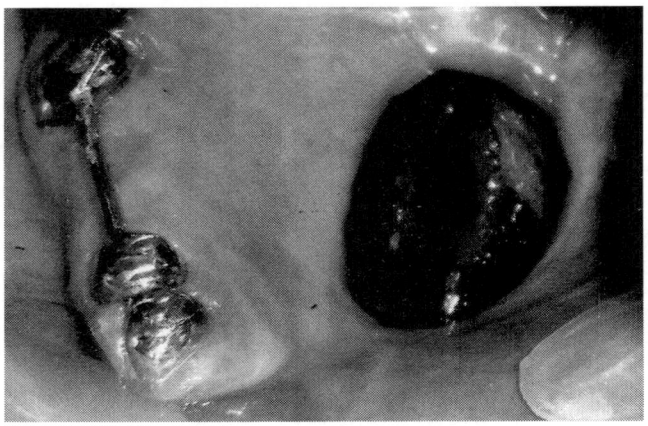

Fig- Bar & crown assembly in place

is carried out in usual manner. After removal from the flask the clip attachments will go in the prosthesis. The prosthesis is finished and polished. The retention of the prosthesis can be modified by changing the sleeves lying inside the metal casing of the clip. The salt used for hollowing of the obturator is later removed by making small hole and injecting water through it. After removal of salt the bulb portion is dried and sealed with autopolymerizing resin. Later bulb portion is highly polished. Definitive prosthesis is inserted in patient's mouth so that clip in the prosthesis gets fitted on the metal bar. Retention of the bar and clip attachment is checked and necessary adjustments are made to improve the retention of the final prosthesis.

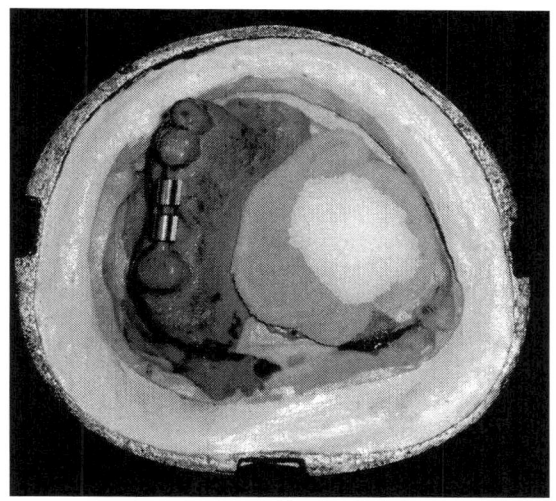

Fig- Processing to fabricate hollow bulb obturator

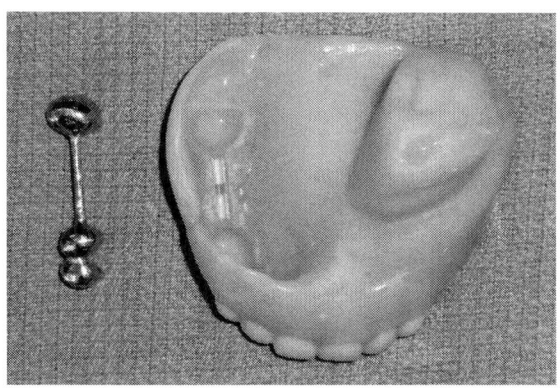

Fig- Metal bar and hollow bulb obturator with clip

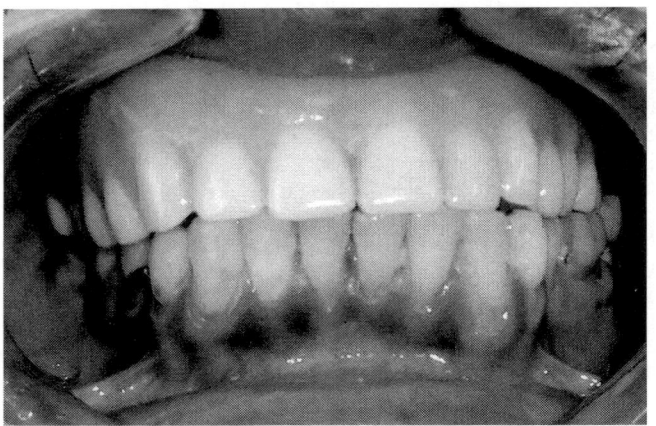

Fig- Final prosthesis in position

After insertion of the prosthesis occlusion is checked with articulating paper and necessary occlusal adjustment is made by selective occlusal grinding.. Speech assessment is carried out two weeks after insertion of the prosthesis. The patient is instructed about proper insertion and removal of the prosthesis. Patient is advised for routine follow up and speech assessment session.

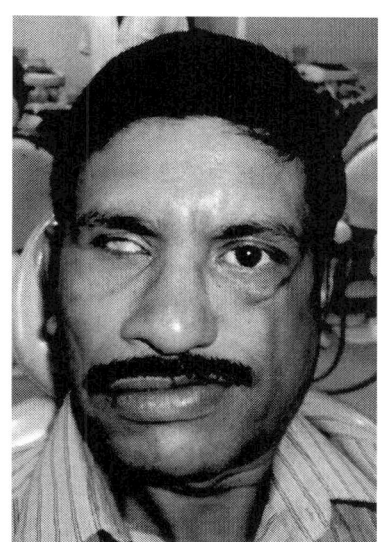

Fig- Before treatment

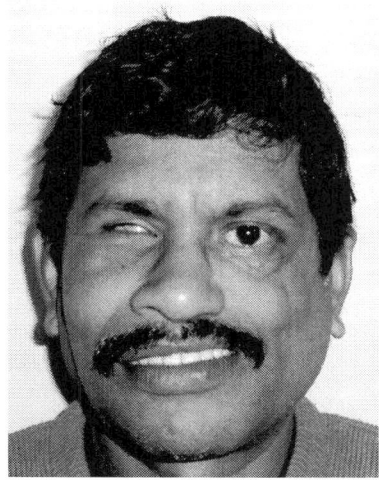

Fig- After treatment

Definitive obturator with cast metal framework

Many factors affect the successful rehabilitation of a maxillectomy patient with obturator prosthesis. Apart from the technique involved in the fabrication of prosthesis the framework design of the obturator is one of the most important factor for retention and support of the prosthesis. Fabrication of definitive obturator with cast metal framework enhances retention as well as stability of the prosthesis. Such metal frameworks makes the prosthesis more rigid so that masticatory performance is very much improved. In all situations, a quadrilateral or tripodal design is favored over a linear design because this allows a more favorable leverage design application that will aid in the support, stabilization, and retention of the prosthesis.

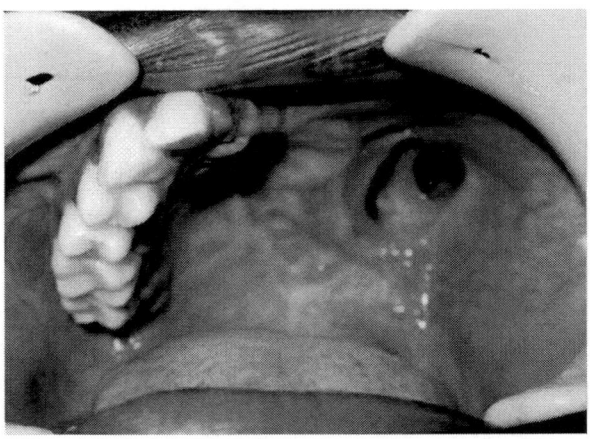

Fig- Post maxillectomy defect

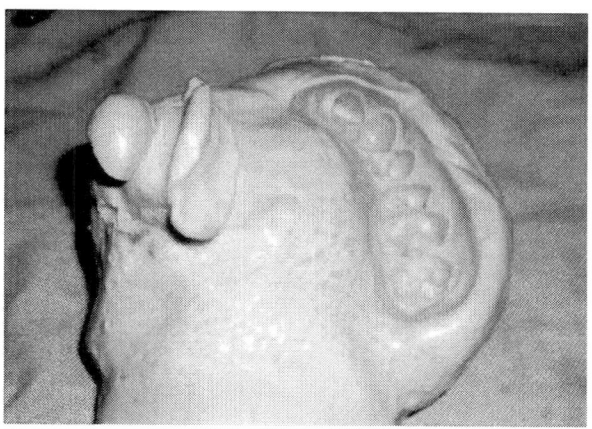

Fig- Final impression of the defect

A special custom tray covering the defect and the remaining teeth is fabricated using auto polymerizing acrylic resin and a uniform wax spacer is given. The defect site is border moulded using high and low fusing compound and retentive holes are made for final impression material. Final impression is made with suitable elastic impression material after all the necessary mouth preparation has been made. The impression is poured in dental stone. A master cast is obtained. The master cast is blocked out properly to prevent duplication of unrequired undercuts and duplication is done using reversible hydrocolloid material. The duplicate model is obtained by pouring it in suitable investment m,aterial and it is called as refractory cast. A frame work for obturator is designed and fabricated with suitable pattern wax on the refractory cast.

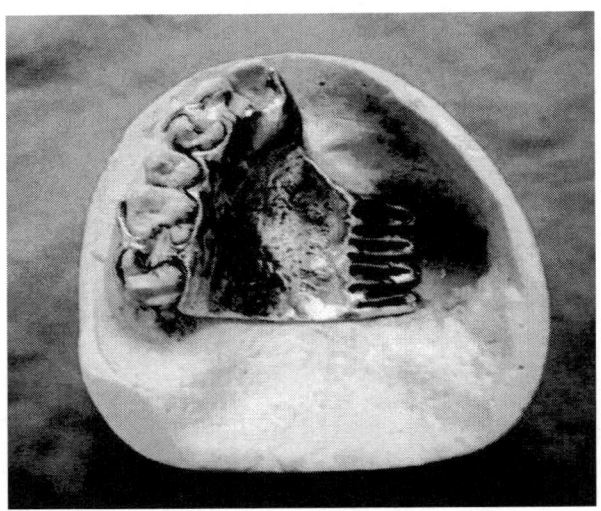

Fig- Cast metal framework

The wax pattern for the framework is invested along with the refractory cast in a suitable investment material. The wax pattern is cast in Co-Cr alloy by the conventional method and the frame work is finished and polished. After finishing and polishing a metal try-in of the framework is done. The framework should be checked for proper fit, retention and stability of the metal framework. Necessary adjustments should be made during this step. During try in the framework should be checked for any interferences by placing in it's place in the oral cavity.

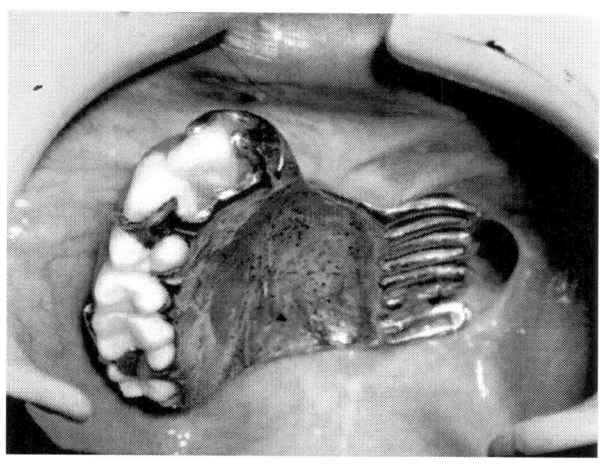

Fig- Try in of the metal framework

. Occlusal rim is fabricated on the metal framework. A jaw relation record is made with the help of modeling and soft carding wax. The master cast is mounted on a three point articulator. After teeth arrangement, try in is done. Esthetics should be checked for better treatment outcome. Speech assessment should be carried out by speech pathologist at this stage. Again the framework is checked for any interference after placing on the master cast. Again final wax up of the trial denture is done on the master cast and it wa\\is flasked in the maxillofacial prosthesis flasks. Dewaxing procedure is carried out. Hollowing of the bulb is advocated depending on the size and depth of the defect.

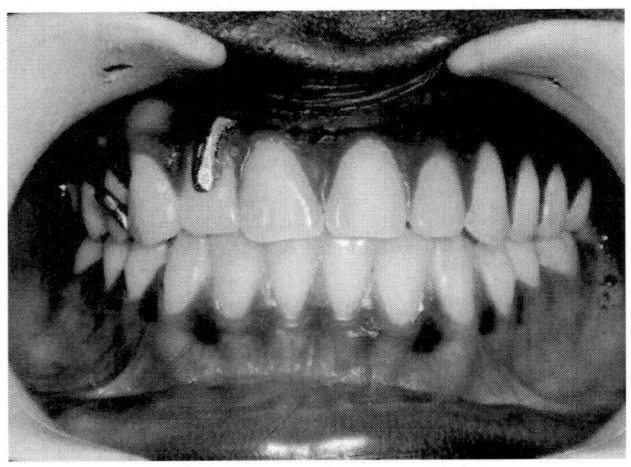

Fig- Try in of the waxed prosthesis

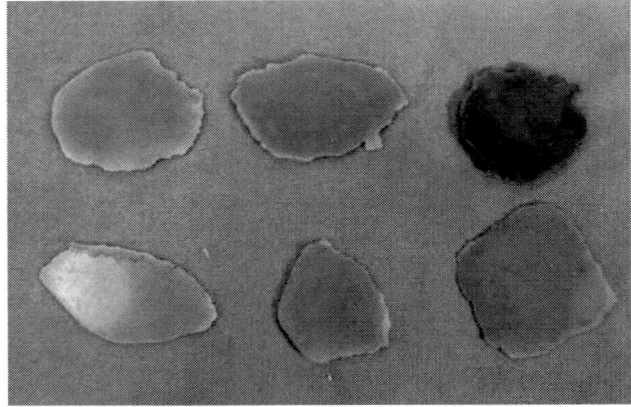

Fig- Custom shade preparation for characterization

Characterization is done using different stains before final heat cure resin packing of the obturator for more natural appearance of the prosthesis. Characterization of the prosthesis with different stains helps to give life like appearance and improves esthetics of the patient. Characterization plays more important role in case of partial prosthesis. The characterization procedure makes the prosthesis to appear more normal. After try in the prosthesis is invested in the flask.

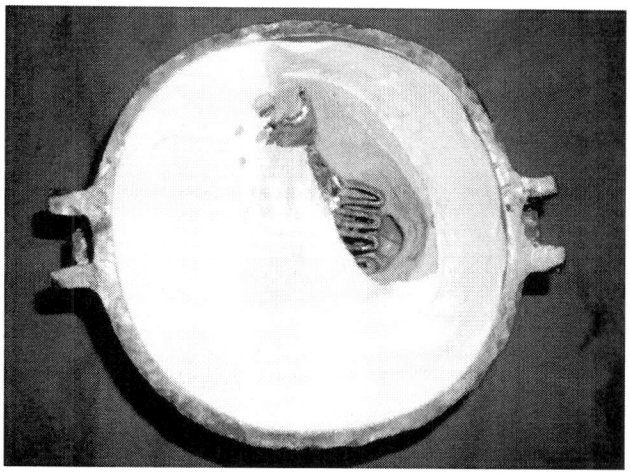

Fig- Metal framework after dewaxing

Heat cure resin is then packed and flasks were closed properly and clamped. This unit is subjected to the regular curing cycle. After processing the prosthesis is trimmed, finished, polished. It is inserted in to the patient's mouth after minor corrections. The prosthesis is then removed and rechecked for proper seating of the components. Post insertion follow-up and patient care are carried out for a period of one year.

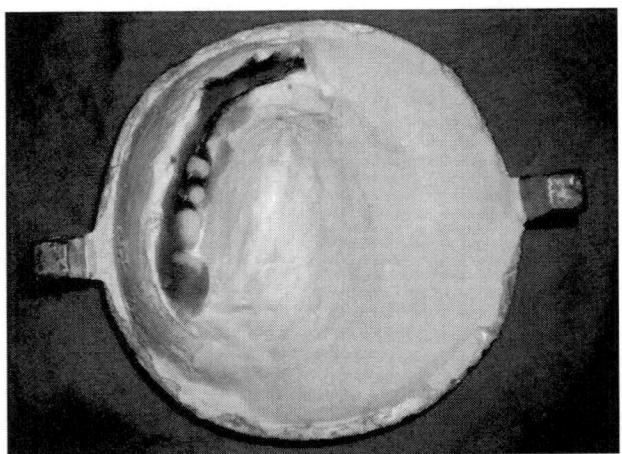

Fig- Characterization done to simulate gingival pigmentation

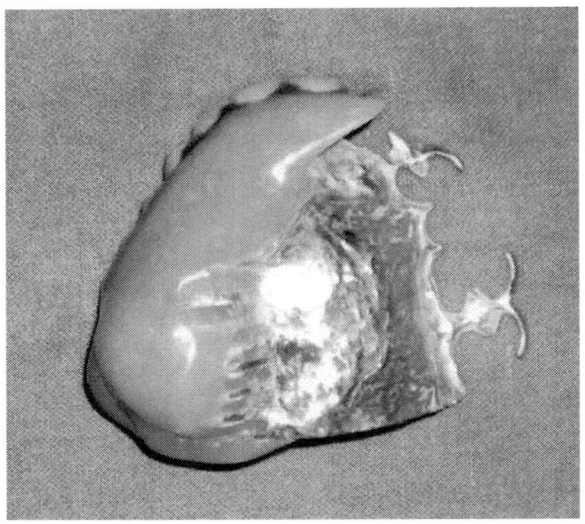

Fig- Final Prosthesis

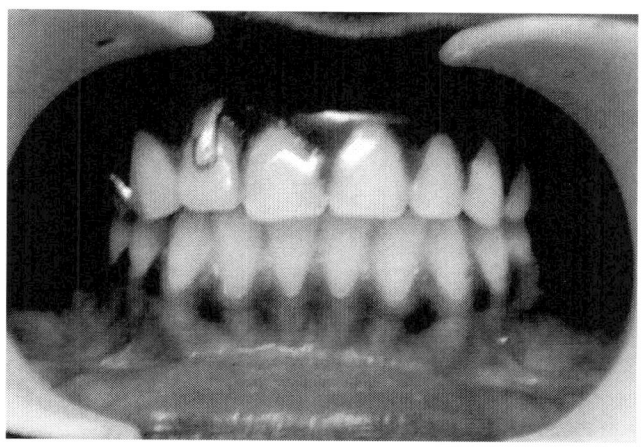

Fig- Final prosthesis in position

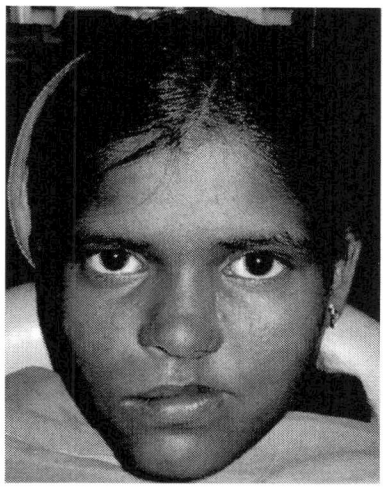

Fig- Before treatment

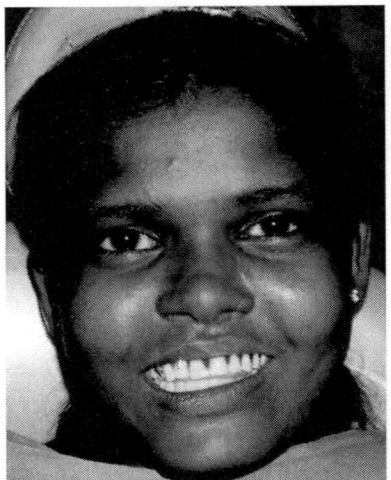

Fig- After treatment

During prosthodontic rehabilitation the support can be achieved from within the defect and remaining structures. Retention can be gained from the non-resected tissue, scars and bony undercuts by conventional and unconventional means.The pre-surgical treatment planning is of immense importance not only for the patient but also for the success of the surgical procedure and prosthesis. Small defects about 3 cm or less can be easily reconstructed by surgery but larger defects pose serious problems after surgical repair making it inefficient to support any prosthesis. In the light of uncertainty a definitive prosthetic restoration is the choice of treatment. Proper designing and fabrication of the definitive obturator prosthesis is very imperative. If the prosthesis is not appropriately planned and constructed it may lead to unfavorable consequences such as pathological changes in supporting tissues due to exertion of disparaging forces. On the other hand movement of the prosthesis will add to additional tissue changes. In diverse clinical circumstances whether in partially dentate or edentulous patients both hard and soft tissues are fundamentally required for the fabrication of a stable and functional prosthesis. The patient shows remarkable improvement in taking food and drinking liquids without any nasal regurgitation. Apart from that speech is very much improved.

Rehabilitation of patients with mandibular defects-

The treatment of malignant tumors associated with floor of the mouth, the tongue mandible, and adjacent structures correspond to a difficult task for the oncosurgeon, radiation oncologist, and maxillofacial prosthodontist in terms of both control of the primary disease and rehabilitation following treatment. Malignant tumor of mandible often necessitates its resection in combination with immense section of the tongue, the floor of the mouth, and the regional lymphatic system. Disabilities resulting from such massive and enblock resections may include impaired speech articulation, complexity in swallowing function, problems with masticatory function, altered mandibular movements, compromised control of salivary secretions, and severe facial disfigurement affecting overall cosmetic appearance.

Obturator prosthesis for mandibular defect

Sometimes resection of mandibular tumors lead to smaller defects in body region if mandible. Such defects if not reconstructed properly remain permanent in the oral cavity. For such defects hygiene maintenance is the major issue which is worsened by food accumulation. It also leads to delayed healing during initial healing period. Fabrication of a prosthesis which will obturate the mandibular defect leads to satisfactory outcome as inconvenience of the patient is rectified.

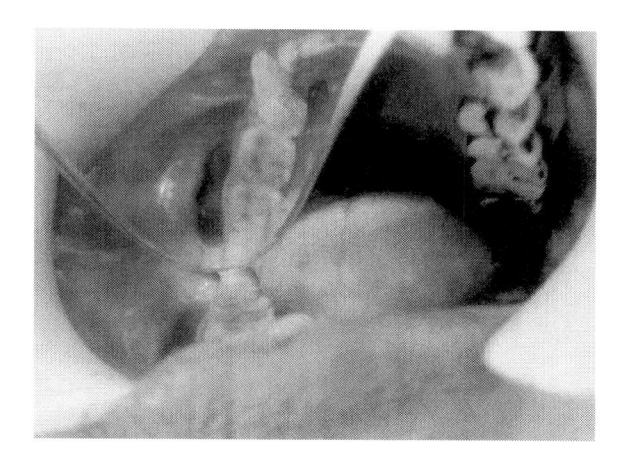

Fig- Mandibular defect

After complete cleaning of the defect impression of the defect is made with suitable elastic impression material. Mould is prepared by pouring that impression and this mould is used for fabrication of obturator prosthesis. It is made hollow by using the hollowing technique. A loop can be attached to hold the prosthesis.

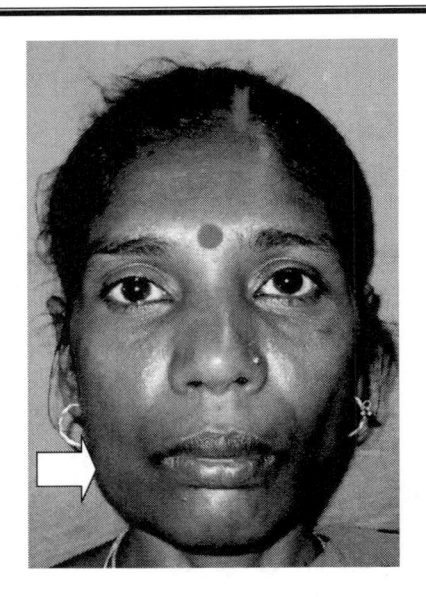

Fig- Extra oral deformity

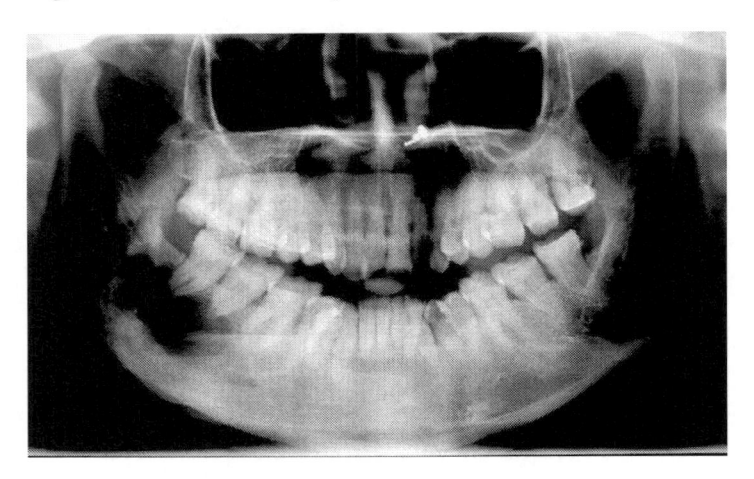

Fig- Orthopantamograph showing defect

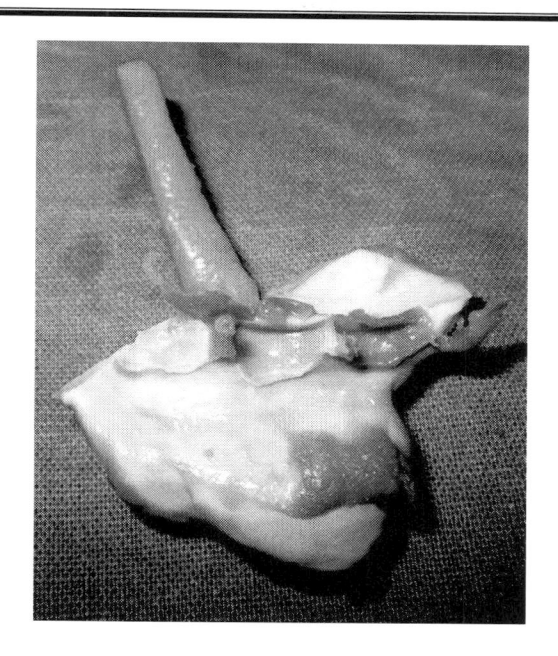

Fig- Final elastomeric impression of the defect

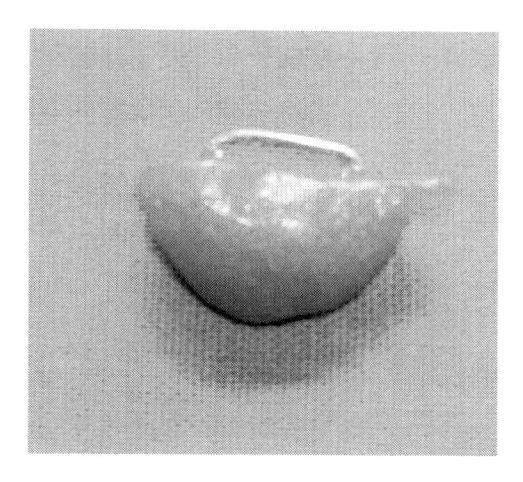

Fig- Final prosthesis

Such kind of prosthesis can be prescribed for the patients who are not mentally prepared for surgical closure of the defect or if surgery is contra indicated due to any general or local ailment of the patient.

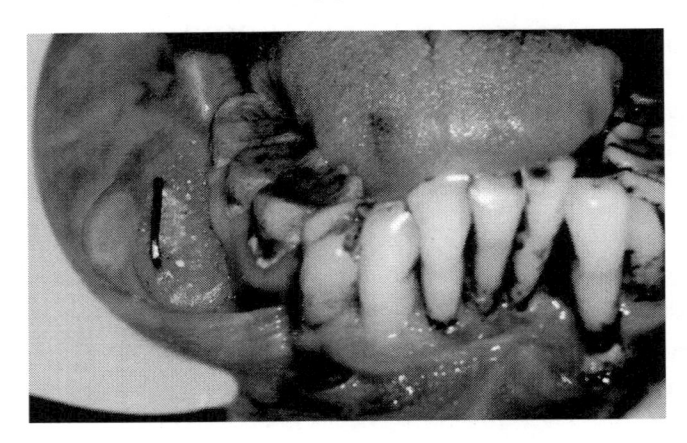

Fig- Final prosthesis in position

Mandibular guide flange prosthesis

As a common observation, the resection of a segment of the mandible without loss of mandibular continuity is usually not as debilitating as a resection that compromises mandibular continuity. Loss of mandibular continuity causes deviation of remaining mandibular segment towards the defect or resected side and rotation of the mandibular occlusal plane inferiorly. Even though immediate mandibular reconstruction intends to re-establish facial symmetry, arch alignment, and stable occlusion, masticatory function often remains compromised. When surgery includes a segmental mandibulectomy, masticatory function is compromised because of muscular imbalance that results from unilateral muscle removal, modified maxillomandibular relationship, and decreased tooth-to-tooth contacts. Although available, osseous and soft tissue free flaps and osseointegrated implants for various reasons may not always be indicated or possible. In such instances, rehabilitation efforts will be challenged and functional outcomes are frequently diminished. Fabrication of guide flange prosthesis helps to guide the residual mandible towards the medial plane so that proper occlusion of remaining teeth and mandibular position can be achieved. Proper designing and utilization of support area is necessary so that the mandibular guidance appliance will not exert excessive forces on the residual mandible and other tissues.

The guide flange prosthesis can be regarded as a guiding type of prosthesis. If the patient can successfully repeat the medio-lateral position, the guide flange prosthesis can habitually be discontinued.

Some patient, however, may carry on for the foreseeable future with a guide flange, and for this reason stress generated to the remaining teeth must then be carefully supervised .

One piece guide bite prosthesis in the maxillary arch is relatively simpler form of treatment from patient point of view. Patient should be advised its regular use immediately after the surgical resection along with other mouth opening exercises.

It is advisable to advocate use of guide flange prosthesis as early as possible after surgery, so that it will guide the muscles and residual mandible in proper position so as to establish intimate occlusion. Delayed use of guide flange prosthesis makes the correction of occlusion very difficult due to contracture in the resected region. If the patient has undergone radiotherapy treatment, then it will worsen the prognosis of treatment outcome with guide bite prosthesis.

Maxillary obturator with guide bite prosthesis

In some cases where mandibular tumor is extensive, it also involves some portion of maxillary arch. Resection of tumor in such cases leads to not only deviation of mandible but also defect in maxillary arch which need to be obturated. For rehabilitation of such patients maxillary obturator with guide bite prosthesis is advocated. Fabrication of two different prostheses will make the treatment awkward, so it advisable to give one piece prosthesis which is combination of maxillary obturator and guide bite prosthesis.

Preservation of teeth is very important in such cases if the patient is undergoing radiotherapy treatment. Maximum retention as well as support of this prosthesis is achieved with the help of maxillary teeth and their supporting structures. For guiding the mandible in proper position preservation of teeth is very significant.

Implant retained prosthesis in mandible reconstructed with free fibula graft.

The composite fibular flap is the preferred donor site for most complex orofacial-mandibular defects. For defects of the lateral mandible that do not involve a significant amount of oral mucosa, the osseous flap may suffice, but the osteocutaneous flap is preferred. The addition of a skin island allows for absolute tension-free intraoral closure that enhances tongue mobility. It also permits monitoring of the otherwise buried flap more effectively. The donor site may be closed directly when less than 4 to 5 cm of skin are included with bone, but split-thickness skin grafting to the site must be considered in the majority of situations.

The fibula osteomyocutaneous flap is also recommended for lateral and symphyseal composite defects that include substantial amounts of intraoral mucosa, tongue, and external skin. As the mucosal defect enlarges, so do the harvested skin paddle requirements. Skin islands 10 to 12 cm wide are available for more extensive defects. A skin graft is necessary to close the donor site.

Rehabilitation of patients with tongue defects-

In the management of carcinoma of tongue total glossectomy is the treatment of choice in advanced stages of lesion i.e. T_3 and T_4. Tongue is one of the crucial anatomical and physiological union for executing essential functions as swallowing, speech and deglutition. Glossectomy is extremely disabling surgical procedure. Postoperatively, patients with total or partial glossectomy have severe functional limitation. Tongue plays an important role in performing three complex functions that require precise neuromuscular co-ordination i.e. mastication, swallowing and speech. Glossectomy is usually of two types.

A) Partial glossectomy
B) Total glossectomy

A] Partial glossectomy defect-

Tongue function is less affected if the resected portion is restored with a free flap. Myocutaneous flaps restore lost bulk and prevent the severe mandibular deviation that occurs in patients whose defects are closed primarily. The residual tongue and flap are centered beneath the palatal structures, permitting the reconstructed tongue to articulate speech phonemes more effectively. Myocutaneous flaps, however, become scarred and immobile and thus limit the mobility of the residual tongue, and speech articulation may remain poor. In contrast, most patients whose tongues are reconstructed with free flaps have the potential of achieving nearly normal speech. The flap restores lost bulk, as does the myocutaneous flap, but it does not become heavily scarred and immobile. Thus, the mobility of the residual tongue is improved dramatically. With speech therapy, the patient learns to manipulate the residual tongue musculature and flap quite effectively, to the point that the quality of speech articulation approaches normal limits in many patients.

Speech and deglutition assessment revealed that the palatal augmentation prosthesis helped the patients with partial glossectomy to improve their speech and deglutition abilities. Palatal augmentation prosthesis also improves appearance and psychological status of the patient. Thus palatal augmentation prosthesis plays important role in rehabilitation of patient who had undergone partial glossectomy by providing adequate function. The patient had satisfactory experience with palatal augmentation prosthesis with a certain degree of comfort and function after six month follow up period.

B] Total glossectomy defect-

Total glossectomy results in severe deficit in speech and deglutition function. Defect in speech articulation leads to loss of speech intelligibility, which can prevent or limit communication. Surgical reconstruction of total glossectomy defects usually involves placement of a musculocutaneous, microvascular free flap to close the defect. Prosthodontic rehabilitation involves fabrication of a mandibular tongue prosthesis after total glossectomy. Rehabilitation of patients with total glossectomy is a very meticulous procedure. Tongue prosthesis with mandibular removable denture helps to overcome this initial reluctance.

The prosthetic tongue may not replace the intricately mobile structure of the tongue which is capable of infinite movements in swallowing and speech, but it can pace the recuperation of patients. A motionless tongue alters the oral cavity sufficiently for the patient to achieve control, over deglutition and speech. Rehabilitation with tongue prosthesis appeared to facilitate the patient in developing compensatory strategies for successfully managing food bolus. It helps to resume social activities, have almost normal diet and converse reasonably in the absence of tongue. The palatal augmentation prosthesis provides convinced degree of comfort and function to the patient. These prostheses can be refined with the use of videofluoroscopy, videotaping, ultrasound, magnetic resonance imaging and electropalatography analysis.

In the deficiency of the tongue and hypoglossal nerve, the laryngeal elevation is affected, thus resulting in changes of acoustic parameters. The tongue or palatal augmentation prosthesis again creates alteration in the vocal tract resulting to changes in the resonating system. Rehabilitation of patient with silicone tongue prosthesis helped the patient to improve diet intake as food is more easily directed into esophagus in a controlled manner and tissues are protected. Speech and deglutition assessment revealed that the artificial tongue prosthesis and palatal augmentation prosthesis facilitated the patient to improve his speech and deglutition abilities. They also improve articulation and resonance leading to better socialization of the patient. Final outcome leads to superior psychological status of the patient. . Patient also feels that his voice is more stable and better resonated, even during continuous speech. Airflow control is achieved due to this prosthesis. . Six months later patient is educated to ingest semisolid food. Patient should attend speech therapy sessions during his regular follow up visits for the next five years. Though there is limitation of physiologic mobility as compared to natural tongue, tongue prosthesis plays significant role in rehabilitation of patient with total glossectomy by providing adequate function.

Pharyngeal Obturator-

A Pharyngeal Obturator Prosthesis also called Speech Aid Prosthesis or Speech Bulb Prosthesis which extends beyond the remaining soft palate as a fixed structure to separate the oropharynx from the nasopharynx. Against it the pharyngeal muscles act to complete the palatophryngeal closure. A pharyngeal speech aid prosthesis is used to separate the nasopharynx and oropharynx during speech and deglutition, and represents a prosthetic solution for palatopharyngeal insufficiency. The conventional prosthesis consists of an oral section composed of a cast partial dental prosthesis framework with a perforated palatal extension to support the obturator section. Patients with acquired defects or congenital malformations of the palate reveal disturbances in speech, including hypernasality, nasal emission, and decreased intelligibility of speech. Apart from that the deglutition is also affected. It is also having effect on the psychological and social status of the patient. Maxillofacial prosthetic treatment can restore the palatopharyngeal integrity to offer the potential for acceptable speech. Pharyngeal obturator is used for this purpose which is also called as speech aid prosthesis.

Surgical resection of neoplastic disease can alter the continuity the soft palate resulting in an acquired defect. The muscles of the palate and pharynx are :- levator veli palatini, tensor veli palatini, palatoglossus, palatopharyngeus, musculus uvulae, the superior, middle, and inferior constrictors, salpingopharyngeus and stylopharyngeus. With the exception of tensor veli palatini, which is supplied by the motor branch of the mandibular division of the trigeminal through the nerve to medial pterygoid, and stylopharyngeus, which is supplied by the glossopharyngeal nerve, the muscles are supplied by the cranial part of the accessory nerve via the pharyngeal plexus.

The palatopharynx is a precisely coordinated valve formed by several muscle groups. At rest the soft palate drapes downwards so that the oral pharynx and nasopharynx are open and coupled to allow for normal breathing through nasal passages. When palatopharyngeal closure is required, the middle one third of the soft palate arcs backward to contact the posterior pharyngeal wall at or above the level of the palatal plane. The lateral pharyngeal walls move medially and posteriorly to contact the margins of the soft palate at or slightly below the level of torus tubarius (medial bulging of the pharyngeal terminus of eustachian tube). Posterior pharyngeal wall may move anteriorly to facilitate contact with elevated soft palate. The level of posterior wall contact is also corresponds with the level of anterior tubercle of atlas (1st cervical vertebra). Complete palatopharyngeal closure is required for normal deglutition and production of some speech sounds (plosives). For vowels and some nasal consonants, the palatopharyngeal port will be open in varying degrees. Palatopharyngeal closure is slightly below the level of the palatal plane up to 8 years of age and is consistently above the level of the palatal plane thereafter. Passavant's pad is most likely to be evident when patient exhibit inadequate palatopharyngeal closure. It may serve as a guide for proper placement of the obturator. The pharyngeal obturator prosthesis does not displace the soft palate but replaces missing portions of the soft palate.

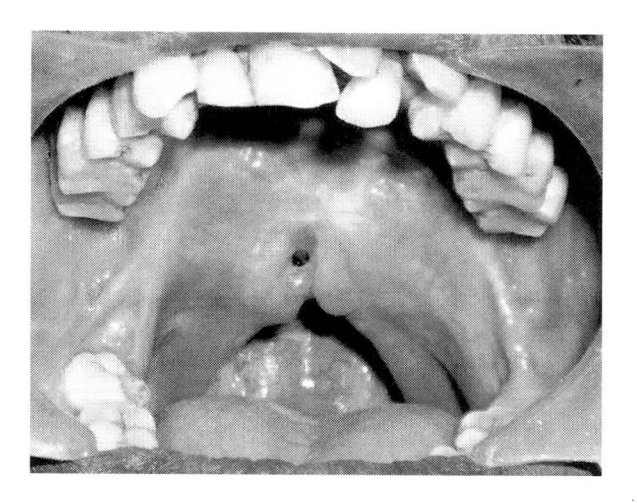

Fig- Pharyngeal defect

A preliminary impression intended to record the defect as much as possible is made. The diagnostic cast is surveyed for framework designing. Design of the metal framework is finalized. Mouth preparations are intended and a final impression is made with polyvinyl siloxane impression material.

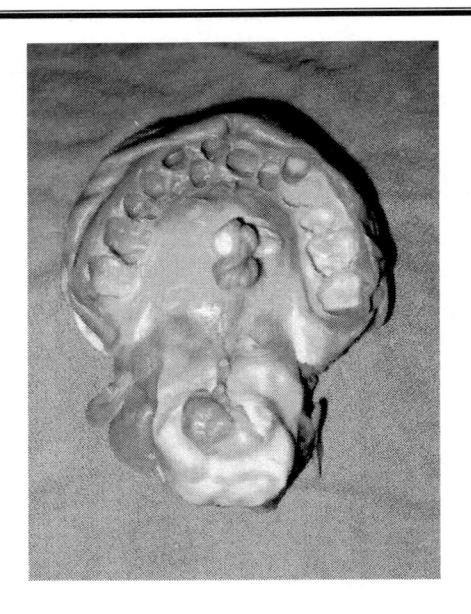

Fig- Impression of oral & pharyngeal section

After surveying of the Master cast, wax pattern is fabricated. The pharyngeal extension is positioned horizontally at the level of palatal plane. After casting and finishing, the framework is tried in patient mouth. Now, the impression for the pharyngeal extension is intended. Initially high fusing compound is added to extend into the defect without contacting the walls of the defect. Low fusing compound is added incrementally after high fusing compound to border mold the pharyngeal space.

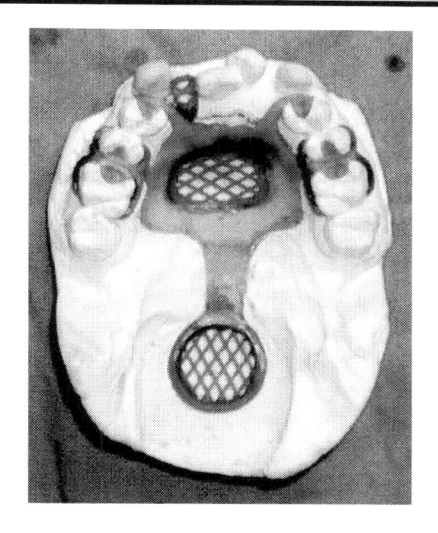

Fig- Wax pattern of metal framework

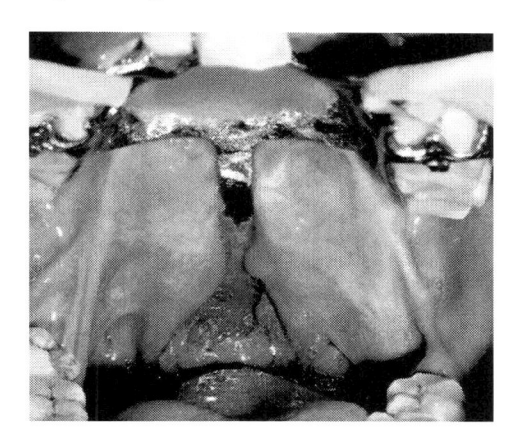

Fig- Functional impression of pharyngeal defect

When the metal framework is inserted in mouth everytime during the impression procedure the patient is instructed to flex the neck fully to achieve contact of the chin to the chest. This movement will establish contact of the posterior aspect of the obturator with the soft tissue covering the dorsal tubercle of the atlas. Lateral aspects of the obturator are formed by rotation and flexion of the neck to achieve chin contact with the right and left shoulder respectively. Once contact is present around the lateral and posterior borders of the modeling compound obturator, there should be absence of air and liquid flow from the oral to the nasal cavities. After slight (0.5-1.0 mm) reduction of the compound, mouth temperature wax is adapted to the modeling compound . The material remains in place for 7-10 minutes and the previous neck flexion and rotary flexion movements are repeated. Difficulties in nasal breathing may necessitate reduction of the lateral aspects of the obturator until breathing is unstrained. Such a reduction of the prosthesis may result in a return of some degree of hypernasality. The inferior portion of the obturator is maintained parallel with the horizontal hard palate if possible. This level will prevent the tongue from dislodging the prosthesis during deglutition.

After completion of the impression, standard dental laboratory procedures are used to transform this portion of the prosthesis into heat cure acrylic resin. Superior portion of the completed obturator prosthesis is slightly convex in shape and highly polished. During delivery prosthesis is applied pressure indicating paste to check if there is any excessive pressure on the soft tissue. The prosthesis is inserted in the patient's mouth and is monitored closely to ensure it did not cause soreness to the soft tissues.

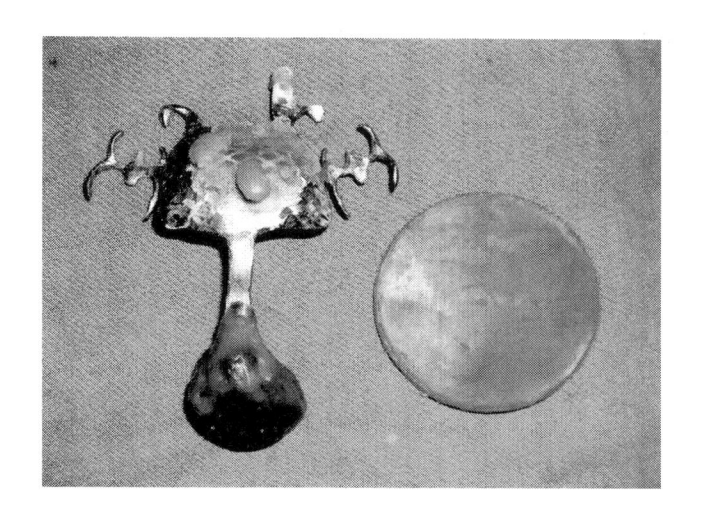

Fig- Final impression of pharyngeal defect

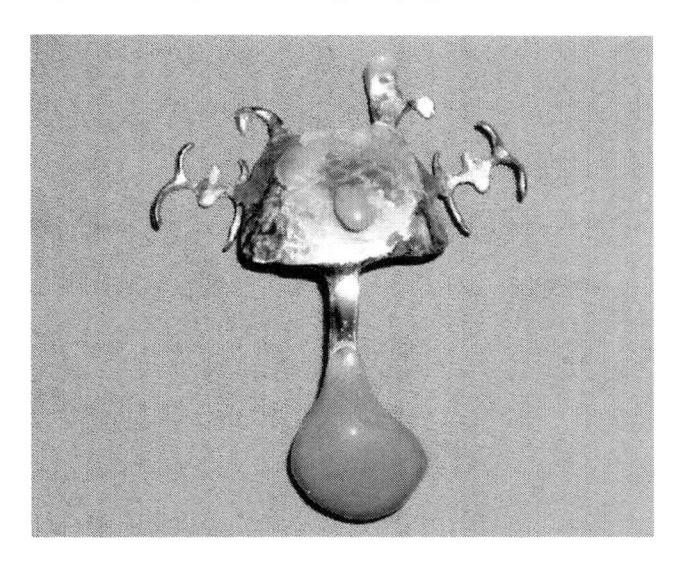

Fig- Final prosthesis

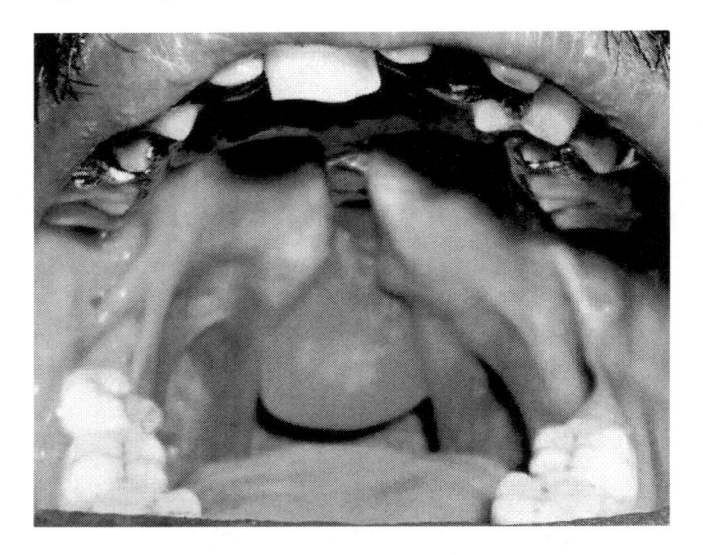

Fig- Final prosthesis in position

Postinsertion instructions are similar to those given to any removable partial denture patient. The patient should be encouraged to remove the obturator for several hours as many patients are reluctant to remove the prosthesis during sleep.

The adequacy of the extension of the prosthesis is confirmed by monitoring-

1. Patient's ability to suck from a glass of water, and water not coming from his nose.

2. Patient's ability to breathe and swallow with ease.

3. A marked improvement in speech. With the patient able to articulate plosive sounds such as b and p.

4. And by verifying the prosthesis with the cephaloradiographs.

5. Over extended prosthesis – chance of gagging.

   During the follow up period there is improvement in the patient's speech and deglutition. Speech therapist may be of assistance to improve speech in case of speech aid prosthesis.

Lip Prosthesis-

Lip prosthesis can be prescribed to the patient with certain lip defects. Lip prosthesis may not fulfill the functional requirements in most of the cases but it is cosmetically very effective to mask the disfigured appearance of the resected lip. In most of the patients lip prosthesis will require retention from the abutment teeth.

Tracheo Esophageal Prosthesis-

Tracheo Esophageal Prosthesis is a device made of medical grade silicone, which is positioned in the "party wall", which is the shared wall between the trachea and the esophagus. The voice prosthesis does not produce voice itself. The purpose of the prosthesis is to allow air to be delivered from the lungs into the esophagus where it is expelled through the mouth. The passage of air as it travels from esophagus to mouth, results in vibration of tissues in the lower pharynx, or throat producing sound which serves as the new voice for laryngectomy patients.

Wax pattern of desired dimensions is fabricated as shown in the figure. Then that wax pattern is invested in the flask. After flasking of the pattern, dewaxing is carried out in a regular manner. After the dewaxing procedure medical grade silicone material is packed in the mould space. After vulcanization of silicone, the Tracheo Esophageal Prosthesis is removed from the flask and finishing polishing is carried out. The prosthesis is inserted in the place and prosthesis hygiene maintenance instructions should be given to the patient.

Nasal Stent-

Internal defects of nose consequence from congenital abnormalities, trauma, tumour excision, and complications of cosmetic or airway enhancement procedures. One of the most widespread reasons for non cosmetic nose surgery is a deviated nasal septum and therefore producing breathing difficulty through nose. But post-surgical scar contracture may lead to the disintegration of airway. Nasal stent is a prosthesis which helps to maintain the patency of nostrils.

Thus prescription of a nasal stent for the patient is indicated during the preliminary period of healing to preserve the patency and contours on the nasal cavity throughout the healing period and consequently preventing the stenosis or collaspe of the airway. The nasal stent is fabricated after the surgery and for the maintenance of the patency of nasal cavity and to grant support to the nasal soft tissues during the preliminary period of healing.

Extra Oral Prosthetic Rehabilitation-

Facial defects may be a consequence of congenital or developmental abnormalities, acquired or accidental traumas, or disfigurements resulting from maxillectomy surgery to resect tumors in the oral or nasal cavity. Extra oral facial defects may affect speech, mastication, quality of life, psychology, and social behavior. In case of extra oral defects along with the disability to perform various functions compromised cosmetic appearance is also a major concern for the patient. As such patients are very much anxious about the unwanted attention of other people due to the unaesthetic facial defect caused by surgical resection of the tumor. Restoration of large facial defects usually requires a facial prosthesis as plastic surgery is not able to produce esthetic outcome in most of the cases. Apart from that surgery is having many drawbacks such as higher treatment cost, general medical condition of the patient, status of blood supply to that particular part of body etc. The prosthesis may be made of silicone, acrylic resin, or a combination of both. Several authors have reported different problems that compromise the serviceability of facial prostheses. These include degradation of the silicone properties, delamination of silicone from the acrylic base, poor simulation of facial expressions due to the rigidity of the retentive acrylic base, and reduced marginal integrity of the facial prosthesis, resulting in open margins. Apart from that silicone materials are more susceptible to cause fungal infection. Acrylic resin bases may cause patient discomfort, cannot engage retentive undercuts, lack movement in facial expressions, and, psychologically, are less acceptable to patients than soft silicone. Attempts have been made to develop new polymeric materials with enhanced mechanical properties, such as high tear strength, low hardness, and a low enough viscosity. It has also been suggested that facial prostheses be fabricated in 3 layers, with silicone rubber as a base material, an inner silicone gel, and a thin outer polymeric coating. Attempts to modify materials to improve an undesirable characteristic have resulted in a concurrent decrease in desirable properties. Materials presently used for facial prostheses are improved, but not ideal. Research is ongoing to develop prostheses fabricated of 2 or more materials laminated and bonded together, each having its own ideal characteristics. So selection of material for prosthetic rehabilitation of extra oral defects will be done according to local tissue conditions, availability of the undercuts, financial condition of the patient etc.

Orbital prosthesis-

Orbital defects caused by surgical resection of the malignancy can be successfully managed by precise prosthodontic treatment. If the lids were retained following orbital exenteration, there is insufficient space for an orbital prosthesis. If an orbital prosthesis is contemplated, they should be removed.

The orbital exenteration defect is close to ideal. The entire contents of the orbit have been removed and the orbital walls lined with skin. However, the position of the eyebrow is somewhat distorted. Osseointegrated implants can also be used for better results of the prosthesis. It plays important role to improve esthetics and psychological status of the patient. Accurate facial impression is essential for the construction of a well-adapted prosthesis.

Successful treatment of the orbital defect will lead the patient to appear in public without fear of attracting unwanted attention. The loss of an eye can be a very traumatic event in a person's life, not only medically, but also emotionally. For many, the face and eyes help represent who they are, and it is common for these patients to feel as if a part of them has been lost. It is the responsibility of ophthalmologists and eye care providers, as they journey with patients through the process of eye removal and artificial eye placement, to provide the best possible functional and cosmetic results. In this way, they can help patients begin to heal medically, and emotionally, as soon as possible. Master cast is made with an improved dental stone. Avoid stones with pigment, for these stones may stain the silicone prosthesis during processing. Select a globe that matches the opposite eye. Prosthesis is checked from several angles. Note that because of contour deficiency on defect side, ocular imbedded in wax is slightly posterior to normal globe. Lines of juncture are placed behind eyeglass frames. Contours associated with margins of the prosthesis must be consistent with the contours of the adjacent skin. The surface texture of sculpting is slightly more prominent than skin. This is so because some detail is lost during processing and extrinsic coloration. Proper surface texture reproduction for an orbital prosthesis is necessary. It is noted that orbital skin folds are carefully reproduced.

Flasking of this wax sculpting is done along with the master cast. Wax flowed into desired undercuts and support areas through a hole made in back of model. Stone will be poured into this opening during first stage of flasking.

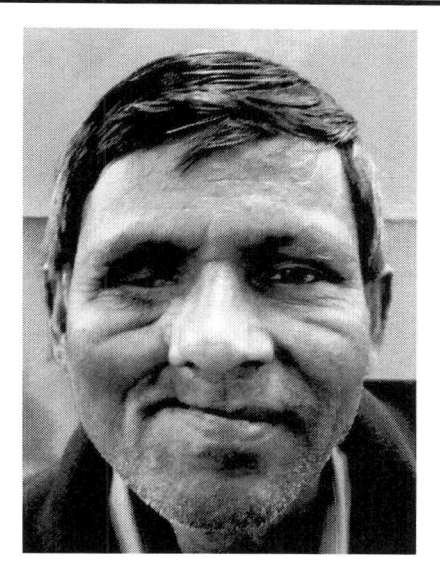

Fig- Before prosthesis insertion

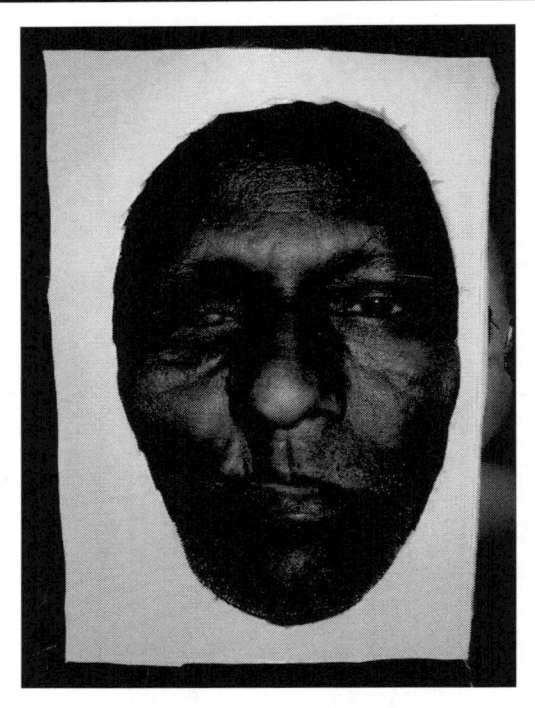

Fig- Customised frame before impression making

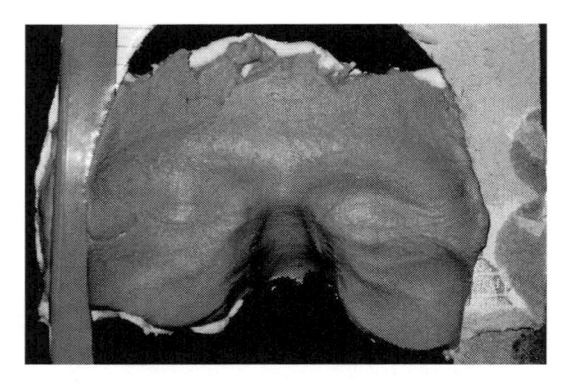

Fig- Impression of the defect

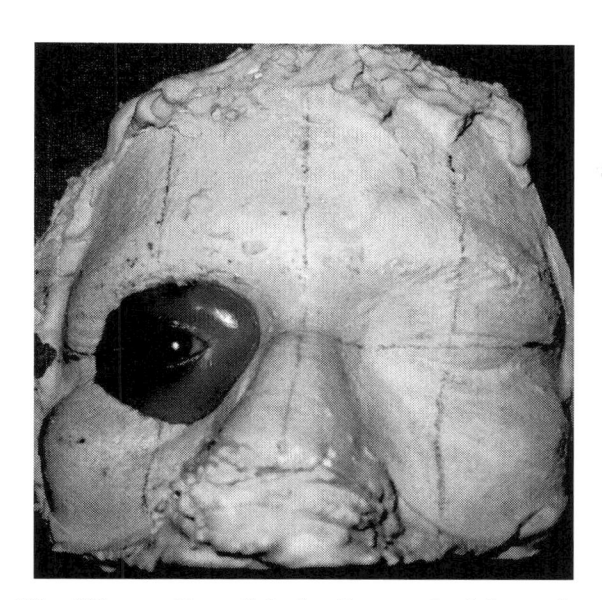

Fig- Wax pattern fabrication on facial moulage

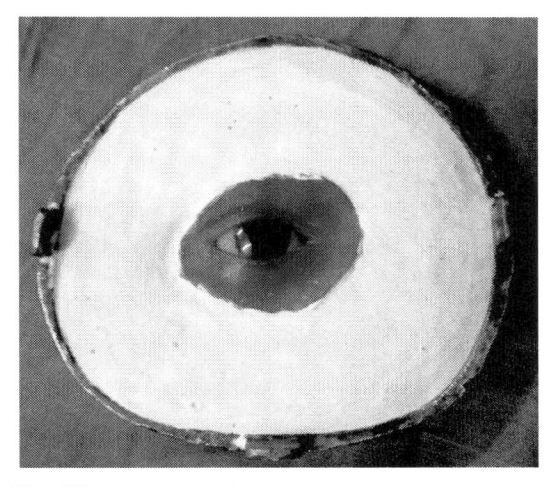

Fig- Wax pattern investment

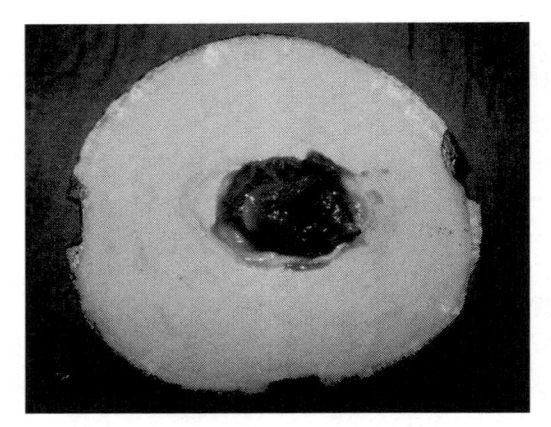

Fig- Silicone packing after dewaxing

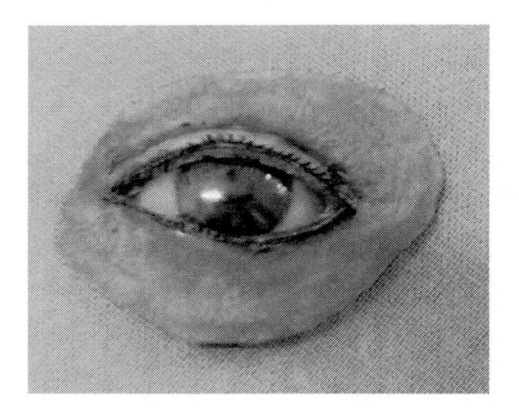

Fig- Final orbital prosthesis

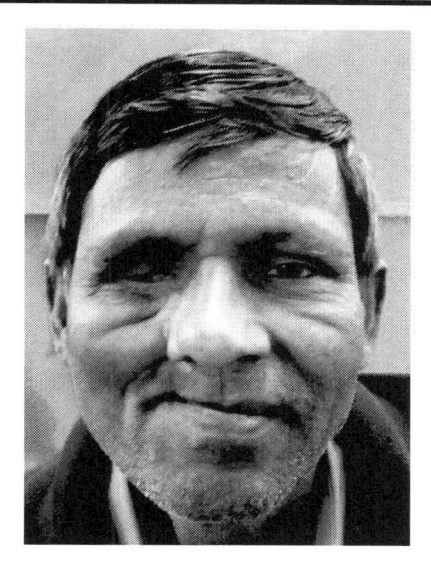

Pre operative view.

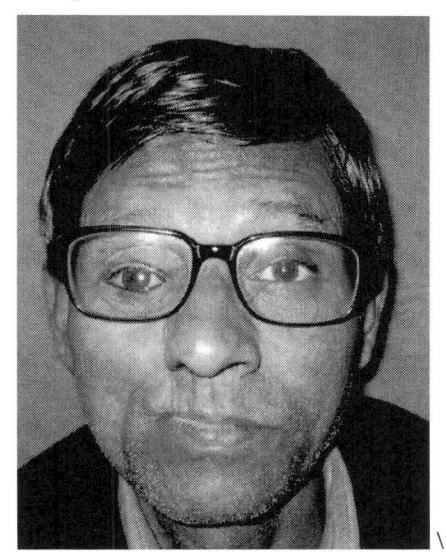

Fig- Final orbital prosthesis in place

The eye glass frames help to hide the margins of orbital prostheses.

Ocular Prosthesis-

The rehabilitating treatment by the placement of ocular prostheses has occupied a significant space in the field of Oral and Maxillofacial Prosthesis. This is mainly because of the great incidence of ocular losses due to pathological reasons or traumatic injuries resulting from physical assault and traffic accidents, which are directly associated with the increasing levels of urban violence observed recently.

The ocular prosthesis, as mentioned previously, is the component of the artificial eye that fits over the orbital implant and sits just behind the eyelids. Eye care professionals known as ocularists are responsible for the fabrication and fitting of ocular prostheses; they are responsible for everything regarding the production of the prosthesis, including creation of the impression, shaping, and painting the prosthesis. Ocularists also instruct the patient on how to place and care for the prosthesis, and they provide long term care for the patient.

Available prostheses are either stock or custom-made prostheses fabricated from either glass or methyl methacrylate. Generally, methyl methacrylate is the preferred product because glass is particularly subject to surface damage and deterioration and usually lasts only about 2 years. Methyl methacrylate is more durable, has a longer life expectancy, and has better tissue compatibility.

Stock, or ready-made, prostheses have their advantages, but they also have a few disadvantages. They are advantageous when time and cost are limited because they can be fabricated rapidly with materials found in any dental office. Additionally, they do not require an artist to complete the painting of the iris and the sclera, saving both time and money. However, most stock prosthesis only come in three sizes and three iris colors. The former is a concern because an improperly fitting prosthesis may not only distort the lid and socket, it could also create an air pocket between the prosthesis and the socket. This may provide a good medium for bacterial overgrowth. The latter is a concern for many patients because often times the iris color of the ready-made prosthesis is noticeably different from the color of their healthy eye, which is aesthetically displeasing. The preferred ocular prosthesis is the custom-made prosthesis, which is fabricated using soft alginate impression material. The material is injected into the eye socket using a "stemmed impression tray." The impression reproduces important anatomical features and is then used to develop a semi-hard wax model. This model can be placed in the socket and modified by either adding or taking volume from the model to further enhance function and cosmetic result. With the use of a corneal-iris button, symmetry of the iris in the palpebral opening and the alignment and plane of the irises in both the artificial eye and the good eye are determined. Correct position of the iris is also ensured by measuring distance from the facial midline and pupillary light reflex in the good eye and duplicating this measurement for the prosthesis.

After the wax model is complete, a glass-stone model is cast and is then used for the fabrication of the final acrylic prosthesis. This prosthesis is given to an artist for completion of the iris, scleral, and conjunctival detail to match the patient's healthy eye. After the painting is complete, the prosthesis is cast in clear resin, cured under heat and pressure, cooled, and then polished. The prosthesis should be tested in the patient's eye for proper fit and aesthetic appearance, and the patient should receive instructions regarding the proper care of the prosthesis.

Auricular prosthesis-

Auricular defects may be congenital or due to postsurgical effect. Contrasting orbital or nasal defects, the tissues in the auricular region are not displaceable, and considerable deformation do not result from postural changes. Therefore, the impression can be obtained with the patient positioned straight, lying on his or her side, or in a supine position. However, condylar movements should be intimately examined, for they may consequence in tissue bed mobility, which can influence marginal placement, tissue coverage, and eventually the retention of the prosthesis. The working cast may need to be lightly sanded in areas of efficient soft tissue mobility to thwart gapping and permit a more intimate prosthesis fit in the condylar area.

Previous to the impression is made, a skin-marking pen may be used to put orientation marks such as the position of the external auditory meatus and the angulation of the long axis of the ear. The defect area is isolated with drapes, cotton is placed in the ear canal, and a appropriate impression material is applied. Adjoining hair should be taped or covered with a water-soluble lubricant or cold cream. Petroleum-based products may hinder with processing of some silicones.

Disposable syringes are useful for depositing impression material into areas with complicated access. Light-bodied polysulfide, polyvinyl siloxane, and irreversible hydrocolloid are suitable impression materials. If irreversible hydrocolloid is used, the addition of 50% more water will improve its flow properties and facilitate the impression procedure.

A backing of quick-setting plaster will provide suitable support for the impression. The plaster backing must be applied in succeeding thin layers to avoid distorting the underlying tissues and the impression. Strips of gauze or wisps of cotton partially embedded within the setting impression material and painted with the appropriate adhesive are used to unite the impression material with the plaster backing.Rehabilitation can be done with implant retained prosthesis for better results. It is having many advantages. Auricular prosthesis will improve esthetics, help to retain spectacles & hearing aids in deaf patients. A prosthetic ear is a simpler process with less risk than surgical reconstruction. It provides an option for patients who are not candidates for surgery. Total auriculectomy defects are easier to restore than partial auriculectomy defects. Partial ear defects are more difficult to restore because of following reasons, blending margins is more difficult and bilateral symmetry may be impossible to restore. Achieving complete adaptation of the anterior margin of an implant-retained auricular prosthesis can be a challenge. Factors such as dynamic facial expressions, mandibular movements, head posture, and facial asymmetry can compromise the integrity of a prosthetic margin. Changes in soft tissue contours associated with these factors can compromise the esthetics of a prosthesis. Conventional solutions to this problem address soft tissue movements at static positions and do not necessarily reflect how the prosthesis will adapt throughout a complete range of motion associated with the mandible and head. The wax sculpting of the ear is positioned on the patient. The sculpture is checked for contour, symmetry with opposite ear and margin placement. A three piece mold is made to facilitate removal of the silicone casting from the mold after processing.

The silicone is mixed, vacuumed to eliminate air bubbles, and injected into the mold. Following polymerization, the ear casting is removed.

The use of the diagnostic wax pattern to plan the appropriate amount of aeration space and tissue relief results in a better environment for the underlying soft tissue. Minimizing prosthetic contact with the underlying tissue can provide a healthier environment for the peri-implant abutment tissue. Adequate relief can reduce the amount of perspiration that a patient may experience and provide better aeration of the tissue underneath the prosthesis. Moreover, minimizing prosthetic contact with the underlying tissue may increase the longevity of the prosthesis because less absorption of sweat and body oils will occur.

Although the concept of cast reduction to achieve complete anterior margin adaptation is not new, this modified technique offers a remedy to the less predictable results experienced with previously proposed arbitrary scoring and sanding techniques. The use of a bur to gauge depth provides for controlled cast reduction based on clinical measurement; thus, the inherent contour of the preauricular tissue can be maintained. A

controlled application of pressure in the anterior margin alone can help achieve an improved esthetic result. The available amount of preauricular soft tissue and the extent of space that must be accommodated can limit the successful application of this technique. The preauricular soft tissue can be identified as the area adjacent to the helix, lobe, and tragus and limited by the TMJ (or where the sideburn of the hairline would normally appear). This area represents approximately 10 mm of anterior extension in the average adult patient. The available amount of preauricular soft tissue varies depending on the patient's anatomy; surgical, traumatic, or developmental compromise; implant location; and whether ideal placement of the auricular prosthesis is possible. Because an equal length of anterior margin extension is needed to cover the space created between the prosthesis and preauricular soft tissue, some extreme positions may not be accommodated by this approach. If the length of the margin exceeds the angle of the mandible, certain jaw movements in the direction toward the prosthesis may cause the margin to 5=[accommodate for every extreme head and mandibular movement, this technique will accommodate for natural postural positions and mandibular movements associated with eating and conversing. The ability to maintain an adaptable anterior margin throughout a complete range of mandible and head movements depends on the flexibility of the material used to fabricate the prosthesis. The prosthetic material that best meets this criterion is silicone. However, silicone loses its flexibility as its thickness increases. The use of lower duramter silicones with greater flexibility may accommodate increased ranges of head and jaw movement.

Auricular prosthesis enhances cosmetic appearance as well as confidence of the patient. Apart from that it supports the spectacles and protects the external auditory meatus from dust and other particulate matter. For cleaning prostheses, the use of water and neutral soap, as well as chlorhexidine, is recommended. As regards care of the adjacent tissues, it is recommended to remove the prosthesis before going to sleep, in addition to ishing the prosthesis receptor tissues with water and neutral soap or with a mixture of hydrogen peroxide and water.

Nasal prosthesis-

Prosthetic management of nasal defects that result from trauma or surgery has been well-documented. Adefinitive nasal prosthesis can reestablish esthetic form and anatomic contours for this type of midfacial defect, often more effectively than by surgical reconstruction. However, a significant period needs to elapse after surgery or traumatic injury before beginning definitive prosthetic treatment to permit adequate soft tissue healing. To provide early rehabilitation, a temporary nasal prosthesis may be considered for these patients. Such a prosthesis can be delivered as soon as 3 to 4 weeks after surgery providing the patient with an improved appearance. This can enable the patient to resume social interactions while permitting easy access

to observe tissue bed changes during healing. Improved materials & shade matching techniques have played important role in rehabilitation of midfacial defects.

Finger prosthesis-

The agony of a physically disabled can be experienced only when one places himself in his shoes. Since aesthetically sound appearance comrade self esteem and confidence, the loss of even one finger produces significant functional deficiency and marked psychological trauma, while the most dexterous individual suffer the greatest degree of impairment.

However, in this era of 21st century, maxillofacial prosthesis has kept pace with recent advances and continuous innovations right from diagnosis, treatment methods, instrumentations, materials and technology to patient centered care.

Silicon elastomers provide additional benefits like superelasticity, retention, pleasing shape, thin margins, life like fingernails, realistic colors in the fabrication of finger prosthesis.

Cranial prosthesis-

Cranial defects caused by trauma or surgery may affect the protective mechanism of the brain. However most cranial defects will have some variable proportion of cosmetic & mechanical aspects & decision regarding cranioplasty must be influenced by the patient's age, prognosis & activity level & specific conditions of the scalp & calvarium. In some patients who may be poor candidates for surgery, an external external prosthesis can be fabricated as an integral component of a wig thereby providing some cosmesis & protection. Materials used for fabrication of cranial prosthesis are usually acrylic resin, titanium, medical grade silicone. Acrylic resin is considered most economical material for cranial prosthesis.

DISCUSSION

Prosthodontic treatment has given a new direction to lead a normal life in patients with postsurgical & congenital defects. It plays manifold roles for the patients from execution of normal physiologic activities to esthetics improvement. Multidisciplinary approach of prosthodontist along with other surgical specialities can definitely improve the life quality of the patient. From a clinical point of view the rehabilitation achieved with this approach outweighs the difficulties in day to day life and high cost treatment modalities for the patient. The challenges faced during constructing a prosthesis are; obtaining a satisfactory working model without tissue compression, proper orientation of the prosthetic portion in harmony with the remaining part, reproducing the contour and anatomy of the tissues, obtaining a satisfactory colour match. The other important issues to be addressed are material and method for prosthesis fabrication and the mode of retention of the prosthesis. To remove the speculations regarding the residual monomer content in the acrylic prosthesis that can elicit tissue reaction, the prosthesis can be stored in water for 3 days before insertion to reduce the residual monomer content. Retention modes for maxillofacial prostheses range from simpler options like using spectacles, resin bonded attachments, magnets, engaging tissue undercuts, and adhesives to extensive options like using osseointegrated Implants[7,8]. The patient visited after every three months for follow up visits. Additionally the patient is advised that the color match depends on the color of their tissues, which may be susceptible to the seasons as well as activity level and environmental temperature. The patient is asked for regular follow-up visits. Multidisciplinary approach of prosthodontist & other specialities can definitely improve the life quality of the patients. Thus the life style as well as the psychologic status can be highly improved with the help of prosthetic rehabilitation.

Summary-

These rehabilitative efforts are more complex and require the efforts of a sophisticated, well-trained, multidisciplinary team of oncologic surgeons, maxillofacial prosthodontists, reconstructive surgeons, speech therapists, social workers, and others. If the prosthesis is not properly designed and constructed it may lead to further pathological changes in tissues. On the other hand movement of the prosthesis will contribute to further tissue changes.

References-

1. Evidence Based Management of cancers in India -2012 Tata Memorial Centre.
2. Clinical maxillofacial prosthetics. Thomas taylor.
3. American Joint Committee on Cancer. AJCC cancer staging manual. 5th ed. Philadelphia: Lippincott-Raven Publishers; 1998. p. 31-9.
4. Maxillofacial rehabilitation, Prosthodontic & surgical considerations. John Beumer III, St. Louis, Toronto, London 1979.
5. DeVan MM. The role of the oral surgeon in prosthodontics. Oral Surg Oral Med Oral Pathol. 1966;22(4): 456-465.
6. McCracken's Removable Partial Prosthodontics. 11th Edition.
7. Prosthodontic principles in the framework design of maxillary obturator prosthesis. . J Prosthet Dent 2005; 93:405-11.
8. Aramany M.A. Basic principles of obturators design for partially edentulous patients. Part I classification . J Prosthet Dent 1978; 40:554-7.
9. Salibian AH, Allison GR, Rappaport I, Krugman ME, McMicken BL, Etchepare TL. Total and subtotal glossectomy: function after microvascular reconstruction. Plast Reconstr Surg 1990;85:513-24.
10. Urken ML, Moscoso JF, Lawson W, Biller HF. A systematic approach to functional reconstruction of the oral cavity following

partial and total glossectomy. Arch Otolaryngol Head Neck Surg 1994;120:589-601.

11. Appleton & Machin. Working with oral cancer. Oxan, UK: Winslow Press Ltd; 1995. pp15.

12. Weber RS, Ohlms L, Bowman J, Jacob R, Goepfert H. Functional results after total or near total glossectomy with laryngeal preservation. Arch Otolaryngol Head Neck Surg 1991;117:512-5.

13. DJ Moore. Glossectomy rehabilitation by mandibular tongue prosthesis. J Prosthet Dent 1972;28:429-33.

14. Skelly M, Glossectomy Speech Rehabilitation. New York: Thomas Publishers; 1973. p49.

15. Kaplan P. Immediate rehabilitation after total glossectomy: A clinical report. J Prosth Dent 1993; 69: 462-463.

16. Kharade PP, Sharma S. Simple method of fabrication & characterization of cast partial framework obturator for life like appearance- A case report. Gen Dent. 2013; 61(6):42-5.

17. Tobey E, Lincks J. Acoustic analysis of speech changes after maxillectomy and prosthodontic management. J Prosthet Dent 1989;18:323-334.

18. Plank D, Weinberg B, Chalian V. Evaluation of speech following prosthetic obturation of surgically acquired maxillary defects. J Prosthet Dent1981;45:626-638.

19. Rieger J, Wolfaardt J, Seikaly HJ, Jha N. Speech outcomes in patients rehabilitated with maxillary obturator prosthesis after maxillectomy: A prospective study. Int J Prosthodont 2002;15:139-144.
20. Sullivan M, Gaebler C, Beukelman D, et al. Impact of palatal prosthodontic intervention on communication performance of patient's maxillectomy defects: A multilevel outcome study. Head Neck 2002;24:530-538.
21. Salibian AH, Allison GR, Rappaport I, Krugman ME, McMicken BL, Etchepare TL. Total and subtotal glossectomy: function after microvascular reconstruction. Plast Reconstr Surg 1990;85:513-24.
22. Urken ML, Moscoso JF, Lawson W, Biller HF. A systematic approach to functional reconstruction of the oral cavity following partial and total glossectomy. Arch Otolaryngol Head Neck Surg 1994;120:589-601.
23. Appleton & Machin. Working with oral cancer. Oxan, UK: Winslow Press Ltd; 1995. pp15.
24. Weber RS, Ohlms L, Bowman J, Jacob R, Goepfert H. Functional results after total or near total glossectomy with laryngeal preservation. Arch Otolaryngol Head Neck Surg 1991;117:512-5.
25. DJ Moore. Glossectomy rehabilitation by mandibular tongue prosthesis. J Prosthet Dent 1972;28:429-33.
26. Skelly M, Glossectomy Speech Rehabilitation. New York: Thomas Publishers; 1973. p49.
27. Kaplan P. Immediate rehabilitation after total glossectomy: A clinical report. J Prosth Dent 1993; 69: 462-463.

28. American Joint Committee on Cancer. AJCC cancer staging manual. 5th ed. Philadelphia: Lippincott-Raven Publishers; 1998. p. 31-9.
29. Izdebski K, Ross J. C,. Roberts W. L, and De Boie R. G. An interim prosthesis for the glossectomy patient. J Prosthet Dent 1987;57:608-11.
30. Gurmit Kaur Bachher, Kanchan Dholam. Long term rehabilitation of a total glossectomy patient. The Journal of Indian Prosthodontic Society 09/2010; 10(3):194-6.
31. Jooste CH (1984) A method of orienting the ocular portion of an auricular prosthesis. J Prosthet Dent 51:380–382.
32. Jebreil K (1980) Acceptability of auricular prostheses. J Prosthet Dent 43:82–85.
33. Aramany MA. Basic principles of obturator design for partially edentulous patients. Part I: classification. J Prosthet Dent 1978;40:554-7.
34. Myers RE, Mitchell DL. A photoelastic study of stress induced by framework design in a maxillary resection. J Prosthet Dent 1989;61: 590-4.
35. Parr GR, Tharp GE, Rahn AO. Prosthodontic principles in the framework design of maxillary obturator prostheses. J Prosthet Dent 1989;62:205-12.
36. Kratochvil FJ, Caputo AA. Photoelastic analysis of pressure on teeth and bone supporting removable partial dentures. J Prosthet Dent 1974;32:52-61.

37. Schwartzman B, Caputo A, Beumer J. Occlusal force transfer by removable partial denture designs for a radical maxillectomy. J Prosthet Dent 1985;54:397-403.

38. Aramany MA. Basic principles of obturator design for partially edentulous patients. Part II: design principles. J Prosthet Dent 1978;40:656-62.

39. Branemark PI, Adell R, Breine U, et al. Intra-osseous anchorage of dental prostheses. I. Experimental studies. Scand J of Plast Reconstr Surg 1969;3:81Y100.

40. Custer, Philip L., Robert H. Kennedy, John J. Woog, Sara A. Kaltreider, and Dale R. Meyer. "Orbital Implants in Enucleation Surgery: a Report by the American Academy of Ophthalmology." Ophthalmology 110 (2003): 2054-2061. OVID.

41. Downes, Richard. "Orbital Implants: Food for Thought." Editorial. Eye 10 (1996): 1-3. OVID.

42. Gonzolez-Candial, Miguel, Maria A. Umana, Carlos Galvez, Ramon Medel, and Eva Ayala. "Comparison Between Motility of Biointegratable and Silicone Orbital Implants." American Journal of Ophthalmology 143 (2006): 711-712. PUBMED.

43. Mengher, Lakbir S., John Lowry, Richard Downes, and S. Ahmad Sadiq. "Integrated Orbital Implants-a Comparison of Hydroxyapatite and Porous Polyethylene Implants." Orbit 27 (2007): 37-40. OVID.

44. Nunnery, William R., John D. Ng, and Kathy J. Hetzler. "Enucleation and Evisceration." In: Spaeth, George, ed. *Ophthalmic Surgery: Principles and Practice* 3rd ed. Philadelphia, PA: Elsevier, 2003. 485-507.

45. Patel, Bhupendra C.K., Nigel A. Sapp, and J. Richard O. Collin. "Cosmetic Coformers." Ophthalmic Surgery & Lasers 28 (1997): 171-173. OVID.

46. Patil, Sanjayagouda B., Roseline Meshramkar, B. H. Naveen, and N.P. Patil. "Ocular Prosthesis: a Brief Review and Fabrication of an Ocular Prosthesis for a Geriatric Patient." Gerodontology 25 (2008): 57-62. OVID.

47. Roman, Fiona. "The History of Artificial Eyes." Editorial. British Journal of Ophthalmology 78 (1994): 222. OVID.

48. Kaydan, Anju, and Soupramanien Sandramouli. "Porous Polyethylene (Medpor) Orbital Implants with Primary Acellular Dermis Patch Grafts." Orbit 27 (2008): 19-23. OVID.

49. American Society of Ocularists. 09 June 2008 <http://www.ocularist.org.

50. Effect of adhesive retention on maxillofacial prosthesis Part I – Skin dressing and solvent monomers. J Prosthet Dent 2000; 84(3):335.

51. Jebreil K (1980) Acceptability of orbital prostheses. J Prosthet Dent 43:82–85.

52. Guttal SS, Patil NP, Nadiger RK, Rachana KB, Dharnendra, Basutkar N (2008) Use of acrylic resin base as an aid in retaining silicone orbital prosthesis. J Indian Prosthodont soc 8:112–115.

53. Dholam KP, Pusalkar HA, Yadav P, Bhirangi PP (2008) Implant retained orbital prosthesis. J Indian Prosthodont soc 8:55–58.

54. Beumer J (1996) Maxillofacial rehabilitation prosthodontic and surgical considerations new edition. MDMI, Inc, Portland.

55. Taylor TD (2000) Clinical Maxillofacial Prosthetics. Quintessence Publishing Company, Chicago.
56. Alice Katz BS, Gold HO (1976) Open-eye impression technique for orbital prostheses. J Prosthet Dent 36:88–94.
57. Pow EHN, McMillan AS (2000) Functional impression technique in the management of an unusual facial defect: a clinical report. J Prosthet Dent 84:458–461.
58. Lemon JC, Okay DJ, Powers JM, Martin JW, Chambers MS (2003) Facial moulage: the effect of a retarder on compressive strength and working and setting times of irreversible hydrocolloid impression material. J Prosthet Dent 90:276–281.
59. Mathews MF, Smith RM, Sutton AJ, Hudson R (2000) The ocular impression: a review of the literature and presentation of an alternate technique. J Prosthodont 9:210–216.
60. Pflughoeft FA, Shearer HH (1971) Fabrication of a plastic facial moulage. J. Prosthet Dent 25:567–571.
61. Driscoll CF, Hughes B, Ostrowski JS (1992) Naturally occurring undercuts in the retention of an interim oculofacial prosthesis. J Prosthet Dent 68:652–654.
62. Cheng AC, Morrison D, Maxymiw WG, Archibald D (1998) Lip prosthesis retained with resin-bonded retentive elements as an option for the restoration of labial defects: a clinical report. J Prosthet Dent 80:143–147.
63. Fredrickson EJ (1958) Mechanical stabilization of difficult maxillofacial appliances. J Prosthet Dent 8:1035–1038.

64. Yoshida K, Takagi A, Tsuboi Y, Bessho K (2008) Modified hygienic epitec system abutment for magnetic retention of orbital prostheses. J Prosthodont 17:219–222.
65. Jorge JH, Giampaolo ET, Machado AL, Vergani CE (2003) Cytotoxicity of denture base acrylic resins: a literature review. J Prosthet Dent 90:190–193.
66. Shifman A (1993) Simplified fabrication of orbital prostheses using posterior attachment for the artificial eye. J Prosthet Dent 69:73–76.
67. Jooste CH (1984) A method of orienting the ocular portion of an orbital prosthesis. J Prosthet Dent 51:380–382.
68. Nusinov NS, McCartney JW, Mitchell DL (1988) Inverted anatomic tracing: a guide to establishing orbital tissue contours for the oculofacial prosthesis. J Prosthet Dent 60:483–485.
69. Mekayarajjananonth T, Salinas TJ, Chambers MS, Lemon JC (2003) A mould-making procedure for multiple orbital prostheses fabrication. J Prosthet Dent 90:97–100.
70. Sullivan M, Casey DM, Alberico R, Litwin A, Schaaf NG (2007) Hyperostosis in an orbital defect with craniofacial implants and open-field magnets: a clinical report. J Prosthet Dent 97:196–199.
71. Tjellström A, Yontchev E, Lindström J, Brånemark PI. Five years' experience with bone-anchored auricular prostheses. Otolaryngol Head Neck Surg 1985;93:366-72.
72. Jacobsson M, Tjellström A, Fine L, Jansson K. An evaluation of auricular prosthesis using osseointegrated implants. Clin Otolaryngol Allied Sci 1992;17:482-6.

73. Karakoca S, Aydin C, Yilmaz H, Bal BT. Survival rates and periimplant soft tissue evaluation of extraoral implants over a mean follow-up period of three years. J Prosthet Dent 2008;100:458-64.
74. Karayazgan B, Gunay Y, Atay A, Noyun F. Facial defects restored with extraoral implant-supported prostheses. J Craniofac Surg 2007;18:1086-90.
75. McKinstry RE. Retention and facial prostheses. In: Fundamentals of facial prosthetics. Arlington: ABI Professional Publications; 1995. p. 27.
76. Tjellström A, Proops D, Granstrom G. Osseointegrated percutaneous titanium implants. In: Maniglia AJ, Stucker FJ, Stepnick DW, Donley S, editors. Surgical reconstruction of the face: nose, midface and anterior skull base. Philadelphia: WB Saunders; 1999. p. 233.
77. Tjellström A. Osseointegrated implants for replacement of absent or defective ears. Clin Plast Surg 1990;17:355-66.
78. Parel SM, Holt GR, Brånemark PI, Tjellström A. Osseointegration and facial prosthetics. Int J Oral Maxillofac Implants 1986;1:27-9.
79. Oliveira MF. Auricular prosthesis. In: Brånemark PI, Tolman DE, editors. Osseointegration in craniofacial reconstruction. Chicago: Quintessence; 1998. p. 213-21.
80. Parel SM. Diminishing dependence on adhesives for retention of facial prostheses. J Prosthet Dent 1980;43:552-60.
81. Bulbulian AH. Facial prosthetics. Springfield (IL): Bannerstone House; 1973. p. 303-4.
82. Nusinov NS, Gay WD. A method for obtaining the reverse image of an ear. J Prosthet Dent 1980;44:68-71.

83. Lemon JC, Chambers MS, Wesley PJ, Martin JW. Technique for fabricating a mirror-image prosthetic ear. J Prosthet Dent 1996;75:292-3.
84. Rahn AO, Boucher LJ. Maxillofacial prosthetics. Philadelphia: WB Saunders; 1970. p. 124.
85. Phillips RW. Skinner's science of dental materials. 7th ed. Philadelphia: WB Saunders; 1973. p. 183-8.
86. Morrow RM, Rudd KD, Rhodes JE. Dental laboratory procedures. Vol. 1. St Louis: CV Mosby; 1986. p. 276-7.
87. Tjellstrom A. Osseointegrated implants for replacement of absent or defective ears. Clin Plast Surg 1990;17:355-66.
88. Watson RM, Coward TJ, Forman GH, Moss JP. Considerations in treatment planning for implant-supported auricular prostheses. Int J Oral Maxillofac Implants. 1993;8:688-94.
89. Tjellstrom A, Jansson K, Branemark PI. Craniofacial defects. In: Worthington P, Branemark P-I, editors. Advanced osseointegration surgery: applications in the maxillofacial region. Carol Stream (IL): Quintessence; 1992. p. 295.
90. P Bhirangi, P Somani, K P Dholam, G K Bachher. Clinical study technical considerations in rehabilitation of an edentulous total glossectomy patient. Int. J Dent. 2012; 2012:125036.
91. Gurmit Kaur Bachher, Kanchan Dholam. Long term rehabilitation of a total glossectomy patient. The Journal of Indian Prosthodontic Society 09/2010; 10(3):194-6.

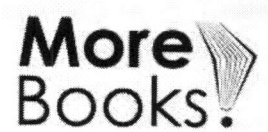

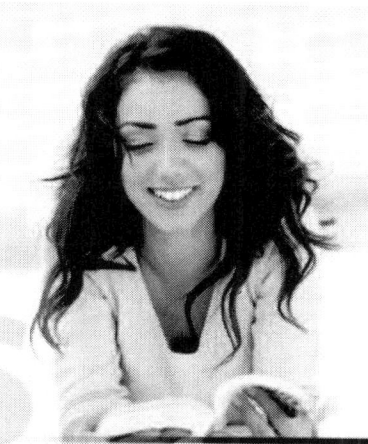

Made in United States
Orlando, FL
24 April 2022

17134950R10057